THE WORKOUT COP-OUT

THE WORKOUT COP-OUT

A Daily Avoidance Guide for Fitness Phobics

Stacey Granger & Dana Mitchell

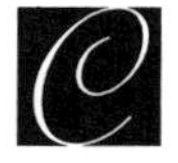

CUMBERLAND HOUSE PUBLISHING
Nashville, Tennessee

Published by Cumberland House Publishing, Inc., 431Harding Industrial Drive, Nashville, TN 37211-3160.

Distributed to the trade by Andrews & McMeel, 4520 Main Street, Kansas City, Missouri, 64111.

Cover and interior design by Gore Studio, Inc.

Library of Congress Cataloging-in-Publication Data

Granger, Stacey, 1969-
The workout cop-out : a daily avoidance guide for fitness phobics / Stacey Granger & Dana Mitchell.
p. cm.
ISBN 1-888952-56-3 (pbk. : alk. paper)
1. Exercise—Humor. 2. Physical fitness—Humor. I. Mitchell, Dana, 1967- . II. Title.
PN6231.E9G73 1997
818'.5402—dc21 97-29580
CIP

Printed in the United States of America
1 2 3 4 5 6 7—02 03 01 00 99 98 97

Thanks to Amber, Ryan, Alicyn, Heather,
and Hailey. Without your endless energy
I would never get any exercise at all.

—Stacey

To Phil—
Thank you for all of your support,
encouragement, and laughter.
You are my best friend.

And to all of the people who have
challenged me to overcome their excuses!

—Dana

Introduction

You step out of the shower, and as you towel off you notice the scale partially hidden beneath the waste basket. Gingerly you step onto the scale and blanch as the numbers continue their upward climb. And even after you deduct, say, 30 percent off the total because your hair is dripping wet, you still find yourself ten pounds over your "ideal" weight. Grumbling, you kick the scale into the closet and swear you're going to shed those unwanted pounds.

Well, such is life in the nineties. America's latest obsession is with eating right, keeping in shape, and working out. But what about those who just *hate* to sweat? And I can't stand not being able to move the day after I work out because even blinking my eyes hurts one muscle group or another that I swore needed to be exercised. And besides, those weights at the gym are *heavy!*

If you're anything like me, you feel as though you lose at least ten pounds just by joining a gym, in so much as I sweat it off by signing the contract giving them half my yearly income and my firstborn child. Then I make the big show of getting in shape by buying all those skimpy work-out clothes (that only look good on those who don't need to work out), going to the gym for two or three weeks, meeting all kinds of new people who use the Stair Master next to mine (mine is set on "Crawl"), and then starting to think of excuses to keep me home the next day.

Then, when I see those same people in the grocery store, I quickly try to hide the bags of chips and cookies in my cart as we swap excuses about why we just haven't been able to make it to the gym. Let's face it: It doesn't matter what excuse we use as long as it keeps us from actually going.

So, in case you ever get stumped for an excuse, here's the perfect book to refer to when you run into your aerobics instructor at the mall or that guy you promised to lift with at the ice-cream parlor. And if you aren't the first to speak, you may find that they are making just as many excuses as you are. Maybe they have this book, too.

—Stacey Granger

To the reader

After working in the health and fitness industry for nearly ten years, I have encountered many different types of people and personalities. Most of them have goals to lose weight, to reduce stress, and to just feel better overall. As the fitness director of an exclusive health club, my job is to give them a sense of well being, direction, and encouragement with an appropriate exercise regime. Easier said than done!

I don't think there is a day that goes by that I don't hear one excuse or another for not coming to the gym to work out. Most of the time they avoid me personally and will leave a message with the front desk personnel: "Tell Dana my kids are sick and I couldn't find a baby-sitter." Two excuses in one.

Family matters are probably the most frequently used excuses I hear. But don't think for one minute that the Fitness Police won't track them down to get them back in the gym within the next day or two. I just tell them that the next time they will have to come up with a better excuse. And they usually do!

The most challenging part of my job, as well as the jobs of other health club professionals, is to help these people overcome their excuses and just do it. After that, seeing the results and feeling the differences will keep them coming back. Again, telling them that they will feel better is easy. Getting them to do it is the challenge.

Getting back into shape is really the number one reason most people join a gym—to lose those extra pounds gained over the holidays or to get their bodies back into last year's swimsuits, for example. But what I don't think people realize is that by regular exercise they will actually be improving their quality of life, and the sooner they start the better. My best method for helping people overcome their excuses so far has been to plant a seed and let them realize it on their own by posing this question: "Do all of your excuses really matter if you don't have your sense of well being and health?"

I usually hear silence and then see them in the gym the very next day.

—Dana Mitchell

THIS BOOK IS FOR YOU IF:

Your definition of a "Sports Drink" is a frosted mug of beer.

•••

The last time you were at your gym was the day you joined.

•••

You consider a trip to the mailbox to be your daily quota of exercise.

•••

You've ever bought a pair of pants a size larger than you wear because you know you'll eventually grow into them.

•••

You think "free weights" are a great bargain giveaway.

•••

You've ever had an allergic reaction to Spandex.

•••

You've ever watched an entire work-out video from the comfort of your own couch.

WORK-OUT APTITUDE TEST

1. A "Sports Drink" is:

a. A high-carbohydrate beverage formulated to replace electrolytes lost during exercise.
b. Any consumable beverage in a plastic bottle with one of those nifty squirter tops.
c. A beer.

2. Free weights are:

a. Dumbells regulated at a specific poundage.
b. Heavy.
c. A great bargain giveaway.

3. A daily quota of exercise is:

a. Twenty minutes or more of cardiovascular aerobic activity.
b. Anything that makes you break out in a sweat, including fighting for the remote control.
c. A trip to the mailbox.

4. You buy a pair of pants that are not your size because:

a. They are too small, but you use them as incentive to lose those extra pounds.
b. They are too big, but you convince yourself you'll eventually grow into them.
c. They were on sale.

5. Weight-lifting is:

a. A way in which to increase muscle tone and strength.
b. A sure way to pull a muscle.
c. Hauling yourself out of your La-Z-Boy.

6. Flexibility exercises are designed to:

a. Increase the range of motion in the muscles and joints.
b. Enhance your ability to bend over and tie your shoe.
c. Increase your ability to out-maneuver your coworkers for the last doughnut in the break room.

7. A sweatband is:

a. A two-inch elastic terry-cloth band worn around the head to prevent perspiration from running into the eyes.
b. The latest fashion statement.
c. Any musical group that drenches the front two rows with their sweat during a concert.

To see the answers, please turn to the back of the book.

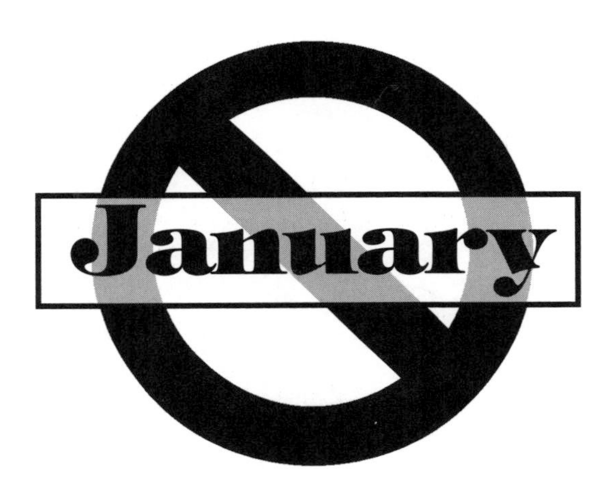

Point

"The beginning of the year is a great time to start working out to shed the extra weight you gained during holiday splurging."

—DANA

Counterpoint

"Exercise is a definite addition to your New Year's resolutions—the ones you aren't planning on keeping anyway!"

—STACEY

NEW YEAR'S DAY

I want to watch the Rose Bowl parade.

It's my year to make the black-eyed peas.

I watched too many bowl games yesterday.

I haven't had my coffee yet.

I have to take down the Christmas tree.

My nose is running.

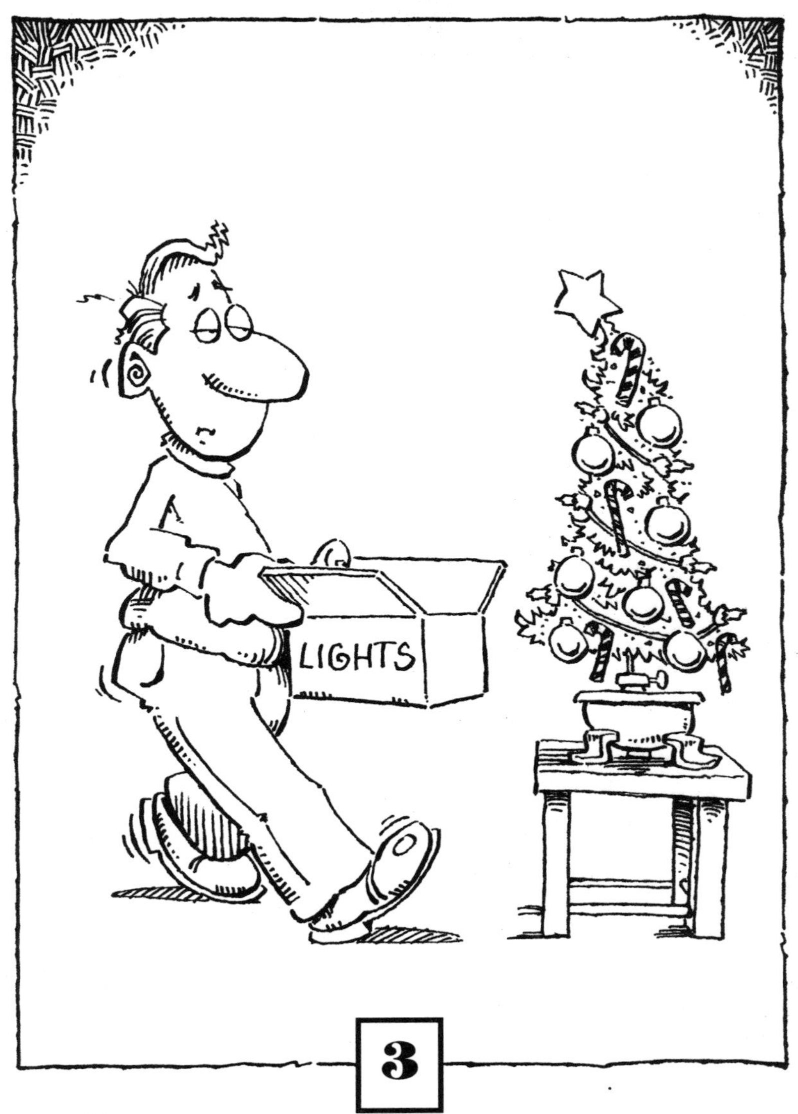

I have to take down the Christmas tree.

I have to salt the sidewalks.

HBO is free this week.

All my friends are overweight.

If I start working out,
I'll have to quit smoking.

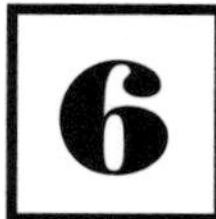

The gym is too crowded;
too many people make me nervous.

I'm waiting for an important call.

I have to take down the Christmas lights.

I forgot to shave my legs.

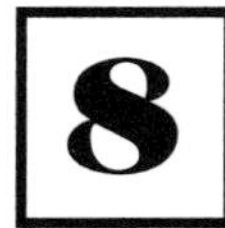

I'm taking the kids sledding tomorrow.

I might miss all the good sales at the mall.

I walked enough at the mall.

I'm having a bad hair day.

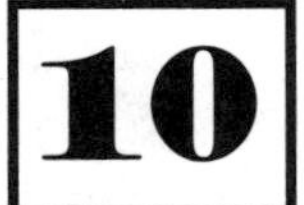

I have a cold.

My car is snowed in in the garage.

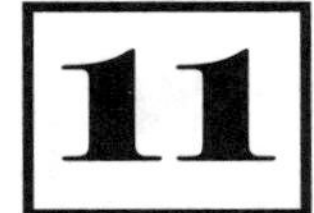

The roads are too icy to go out.

I don't want to weigh less than my wife.

I don't believe in New Year's resolutions.

Exercise gives me gas.

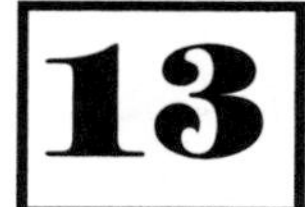

I have to salt the sidewalks.

I just ordered a pizza.

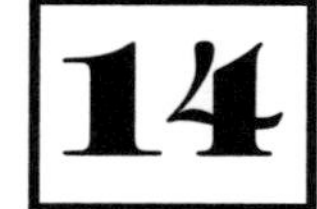

I had my secretary work out for me.

Donuts are free at the coffee shop today.

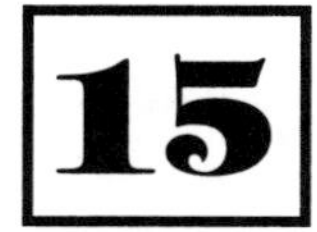

I'll quit eating fast food instead.

I'm proud of my girth.

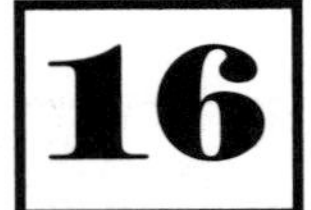

I'm busy reading the next book
in Oprah's book club.

I'll start tomorrow.

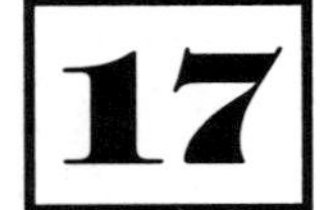

I'm watching Home Shopping Network, and
I don't want to miss a good deal.

If I lose any weight,
my new clothes won't fit.

I feel beauty is only skin deep.

It's snowing.

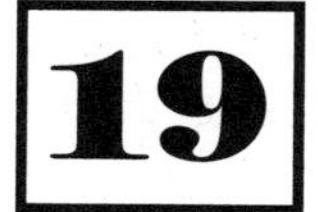

MARTIN LUTHER KING JR. DAY*

I had a dream that I shouldn't work out.

I'm promoting nonviolent activities today.

I have cramps.

There are too many stoplights between my house and the gym.

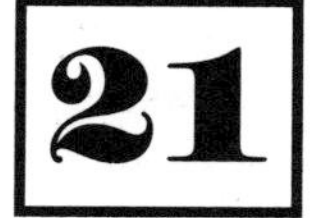

I think I have food poisoning.

I have to go to traffic court.

*Date changes yearly

My sports bra is stretched out.

I'm out of deodorant.

I'm in the middle of a crossword puzzle.

I've heard you can get repetitive stress syndrome from those Ski Masters.

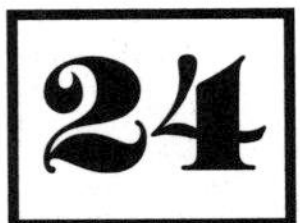

My favorite aerobics instructor quit.

I like being fat.

I look really bad in those skimpy outfits.

I have to shovel out the driveway.

26

Knowing all those naked men are in the locker room next door scares me.

I'm making a snow man with my kids.

27

I'm still cleaning up from the holidays.

I have a hangover.

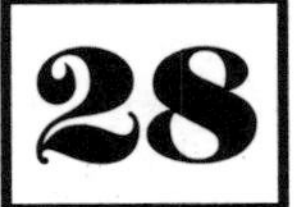

I'm having my hair done.

I'm working on my beard.

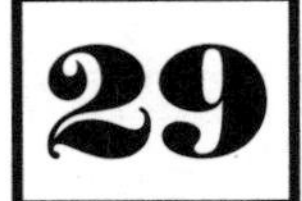

I have no idea where to start.

The car is buried in the snow.

I drink diet soda.

There's a good movie on TV.

I'm going to a basketball game tonight.

I'm not sleeping well lately.

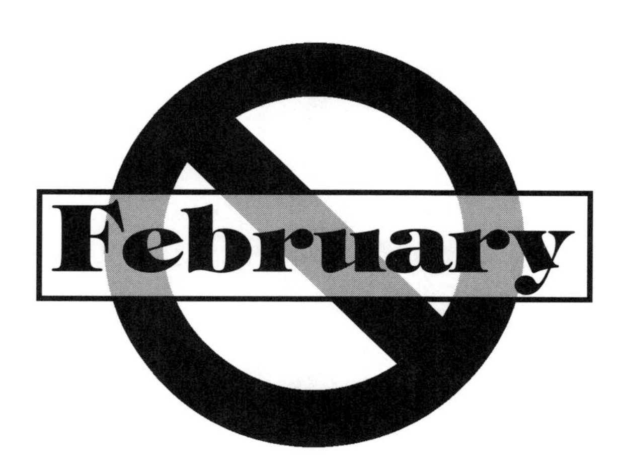

Point

"Don't let bad weather keep you out of the gym. Exercise is great for relieving depression."

—DANA

Counterpoint

"Since February is the shortest month of the year, it won't hurt to put off exercising until March."

—STACEY

The baby is teething.

I have to go on a sales call.

GROUNDHOG DAY

Punxsutawney Phil didn't see his shadow, and I'm depressed.

I didn't see my shadow. I don't need to work out.

I'll smudge my makeup.

I hate to sweat.

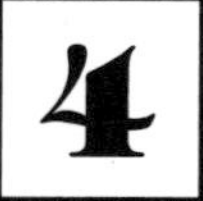

I get enough exercise chasing my kids around.

The power's out.

I just ate.

I haven't eaten.

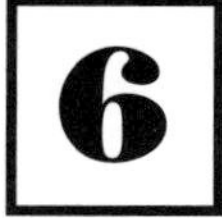

My big toe hurts.

I was really active yesterday.

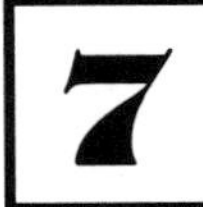

I think I might be pregnant.

I have to get up early.

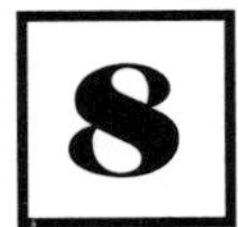

I'm clipping coupons today.

I'm still sore from last week's workout.

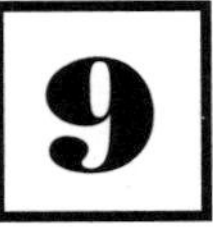

I'm too busy eating my chocolate hearts.

I have to change the oil in my car.

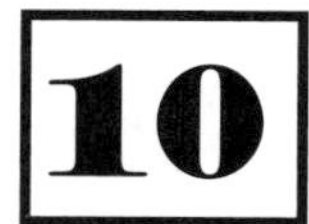

I can't fit into my bodysuit.

I'm surfing "The Web."

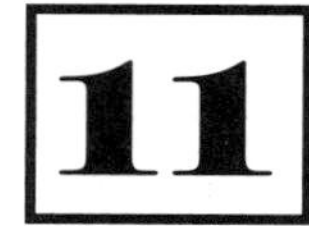

My workout partner is sick.

I have to pay the bills.

LINCOLN'S BIRTHDAY

I've been quarantined.

Four score and seven pounds ago I could get a leotard in my size. I'm not going in a tent.

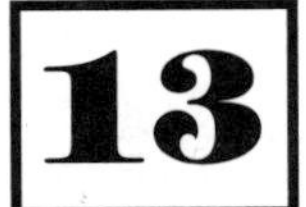

I'm exhausted from all the energy I've spent dreading Valentine's Day.

I have to buy flowers for my wife.

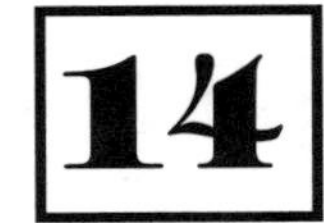

VALENTINE'S DAY

I can't leave the house until my roses have been delivered.

I'll get all the exercise I need throwing candy hearts at the dog.

I dropped my wedding ring down the drain.

I'm waiting for the plumber.

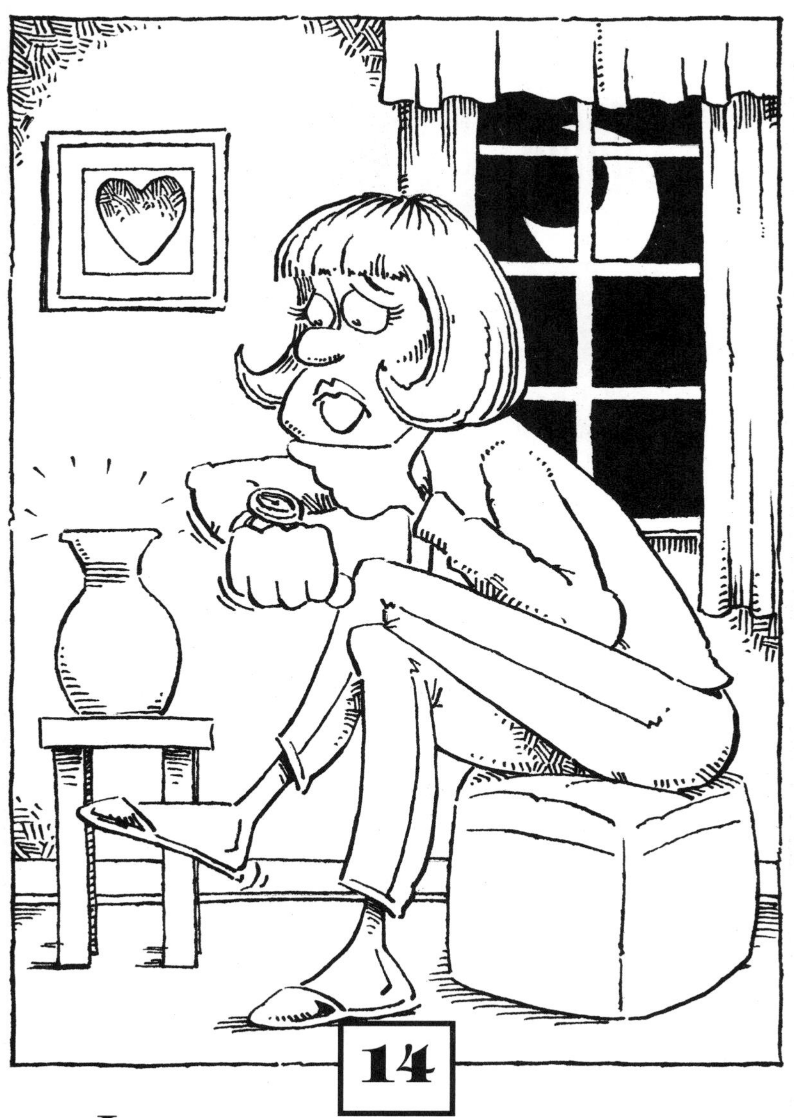

I can't leave the house until my roses have been delivered.

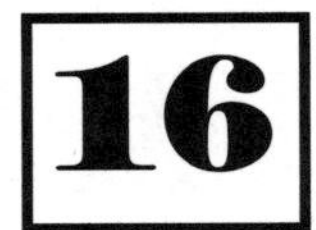

PRESIDENT'S DAY*

It's President's Day, and my kids have the day off.

I haven't cleaned the ice off our sidewalks yet.

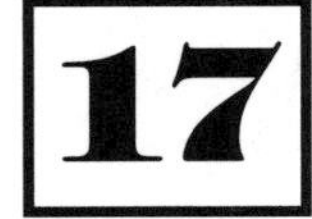

I think I feel spring coming.

I'm intimidated by gyms.

My kids are sick.

I have no one to work out with.

*Date changes yearly

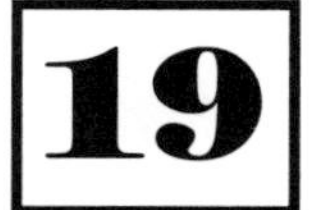

My car's in the shop.

I think I'm going to be busy.

I need to clean the hair out of my brush.

I'm afraid I'll drop the soap in the shower at the gym.

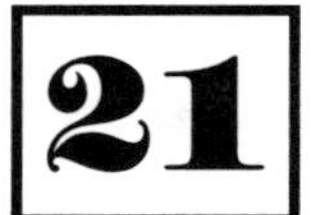

I can't wear my white cross-trainers before Easter.

I'm stopping to smell the flowers today.

WASHINGTON'S BIRTHDAY

I'm baking a pound cake in the shape of the Washington Monument.

I'll just stay home and pit some cherries.

I'm reorganizing my cupboards.

My daughter has a piano lesson.

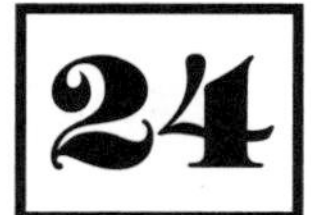

FAT TUESDAY*

Fat Tuesday is my personal holiday. I'm celebrating at the buffet.

I'm planning to go to the Mardi Gras party as a big old slug.

ASH WEDNESDAY*

I'm giving up sweat for Lent.

Okay, I do feel guilty. But I'm still not going to work out.

*Date changes yearly

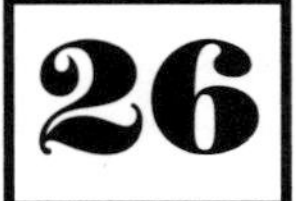

I'll think about it tomorrow.

I had unexpected company.

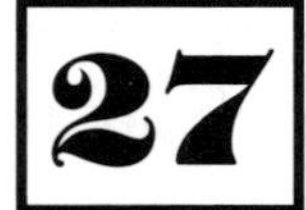

I bit my tongue the last time I worked out.

My wife has been complaining that I'm never home.

The weatherman's predicting a bad storm.

My feet have been smelling really bad.

This day only comes around once every four years.

I'm teaching my old dog new tricks.

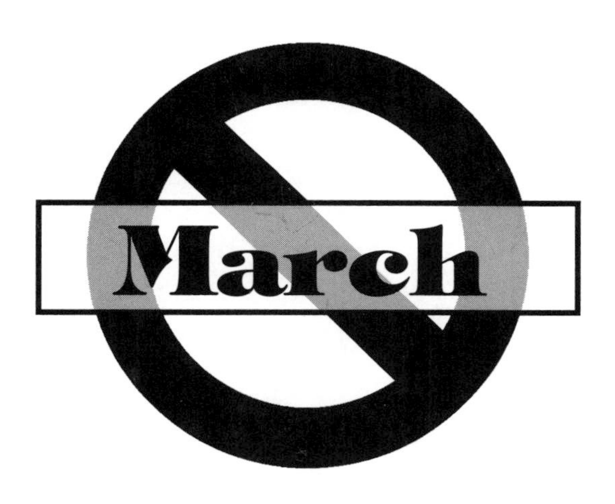

Point

"In like a lamb, out like a lion—that's how you'll feel after a trip to the gym. Exercise will give you more energy as winter slowly drags you down."

—DANA

Counterpoint

"There is still plenty of time before swim-suit season is in full swing."

—STACEY

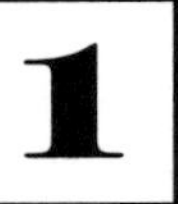

It's family night, and we're going out for burgers.

I'm looking at some real estate.

I got called for jury duty.

I'm a scientist. I work out mentally.

I don't look good in sweat pants.

I have to help my son rehearse for the school play.

I've missed my art class too
many times recently.

Today's my turn to feed the fish.

The locker room smells like sweaty shoes.

If I gain any more weight, I will.

I don't have a thing to wear to the gym.

It's a full moon.

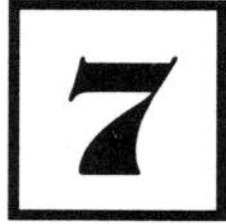

I couldn't find a sitter.

I have arthritis.

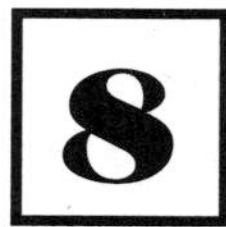

I feel a migraine coming on.

We're leaving on vacation tomorrow.

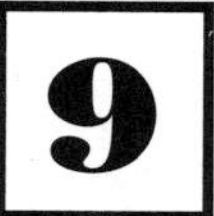

I swear, one of these days
I'm going to do it.

I don't have the right kind of shoes.

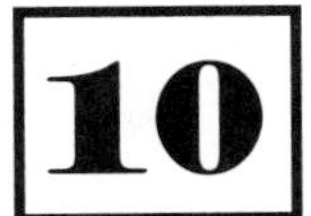

The laundry is piled sky high.

I already have other plans.

12

I'm taking medication.

I don't need an excuse. I'm just lazy.

I have a tummy ache.

I need a nap.

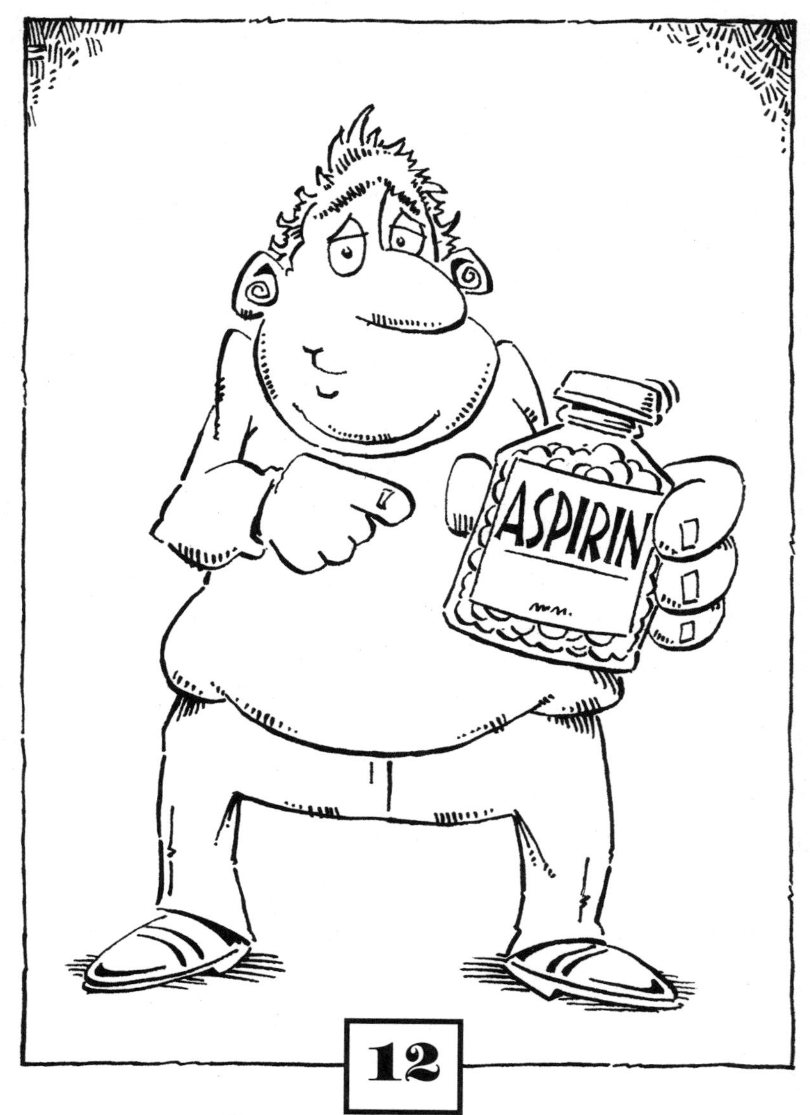

I'm taking medication.

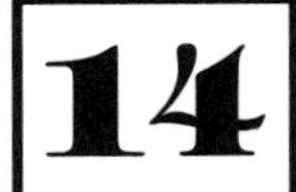

I have a bad back.

I got stuck in traffic.

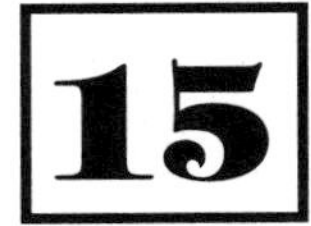

THE IDES OF MARCH

I'm brushing up on my Shakespeare today.

Beware the mood I'll be in if I go
to the gym today.

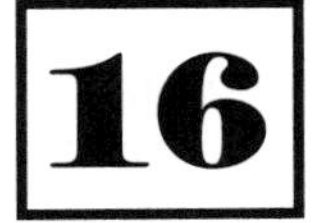

I'm beyond all help.

I'm checking out the back yard
for four-leaf clovers.

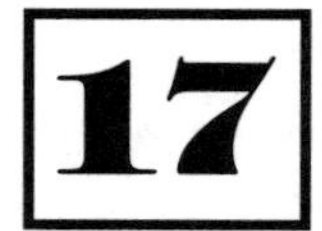

ST PATRICK'S DAY

You've got to be kidding. It's St. Paddy's Day.

I don't have any workout clothes.

I might pull a muscle.

I drank too much green beer yesterday.

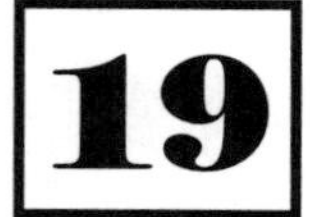

I'm too busy taste-testing the truffles my boyfriend bought for me.

I need to reshingle the roof.

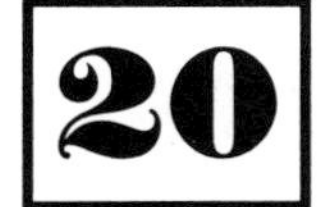

I'm spring cleaning.

I look silly in tights.

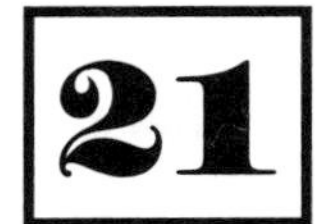

FIRST DAY OF SPRING

I'm worn out from spring cleaning.

It's too windy.

I'm eating fat-free.

I was in an accident.

I have to catch up on the ironing.

The weights make my hands stink.

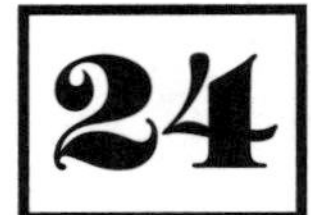

I get a wedgie when I work out.

My secretary's on vacation.

Everyone else is busy, and I don't want to work out alone.

I forgot to set my alarm.

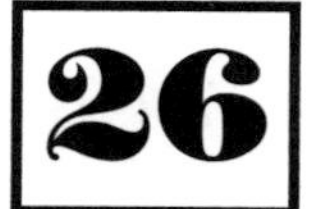

I got a paper cut.

My weight belt is too small.

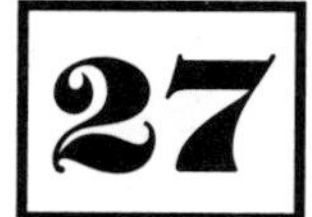

I need to pluck my eyebrows.

I have to help my son with a chemistry project.

I worked all week.

My wife said she'd work out for me.

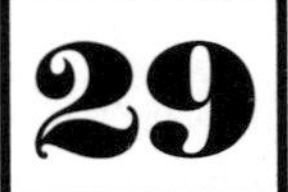

The guys in the gym stink.

My lifting gloves are worn out.

My freezer needs defrosting.

I'm not the ambitious type.

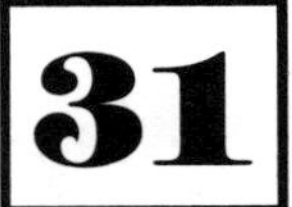

I just put dinner on the table.

I still have whiplash from my accident.

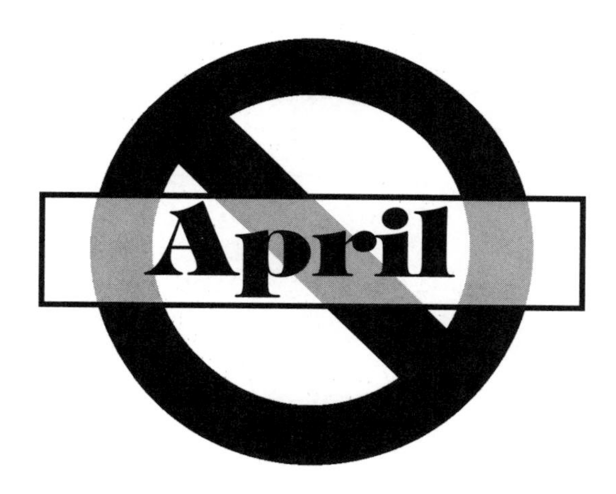

Point

"Spring is a time of new beginnings. Put fitness at the top of your list of priorities."

—DANA

Counterpoint

"All the new summer clothes come out this month. Shopping must come first if you want a good selection."

—STACEY

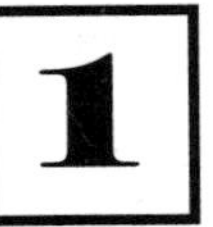

APRIL FOOL'S DAY

The gym burned down.

I'm going to work out today. . . . April Fools!

I'm thinking of running for public office.

I lost the directions to the gym.

I lost track of the time.

I have to unclog the toilet.

My pizza will get cold.

I will right after the spring thaw.

DAYLIGHT SAVINGS TIME*
PALM SUNDAY*

Where does the time go? I won't be able to squeeze in a trip to the gym.

Waving those palm branches around is great aerobic exercise.

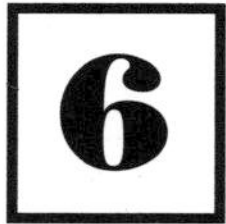

I don't want to get big muscles.

I'd rather watch.

*Date changes yearly

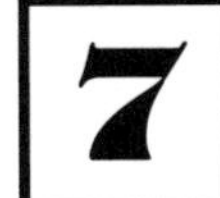

I'm not tan enough.

I've got flat feet.

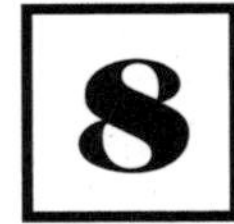

I'm breast feeding.

I have to wash all the windows.

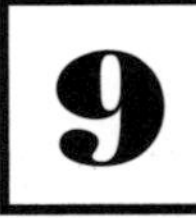

I think I sprained my ankle.

Those thongs are really uncomfortable.

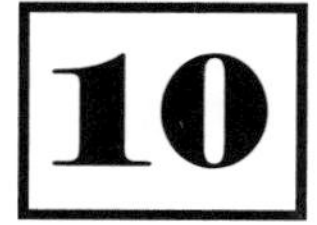

GOOD FRIDAY*

I'm baking a ham. I'll just lift it a couple of extra times.

I've got to think about where I'm going to hide the eggs.

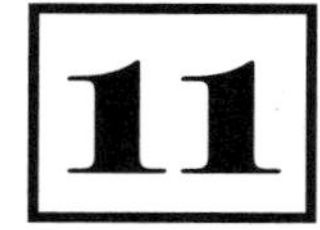

PASSOVER*

I'm taking a pass on exercise.

I'm coloring eggs.

EASTER*

I've got to supervise the egg hunt.

I pulled a hamstring wearing my new white pumps.

*Date changes yearly

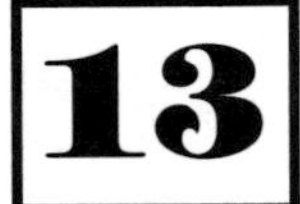

I'm looking for the eggs the kids missed.

I ate too much Easter candy.

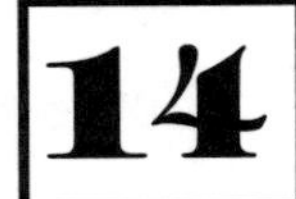

I'm too busy eating jelly beans.

I still haven't finished the big chocolate bunny in my Easter basket.

I'm going to a taxpayers' dessert buffet.

I have a doctor's appointment.

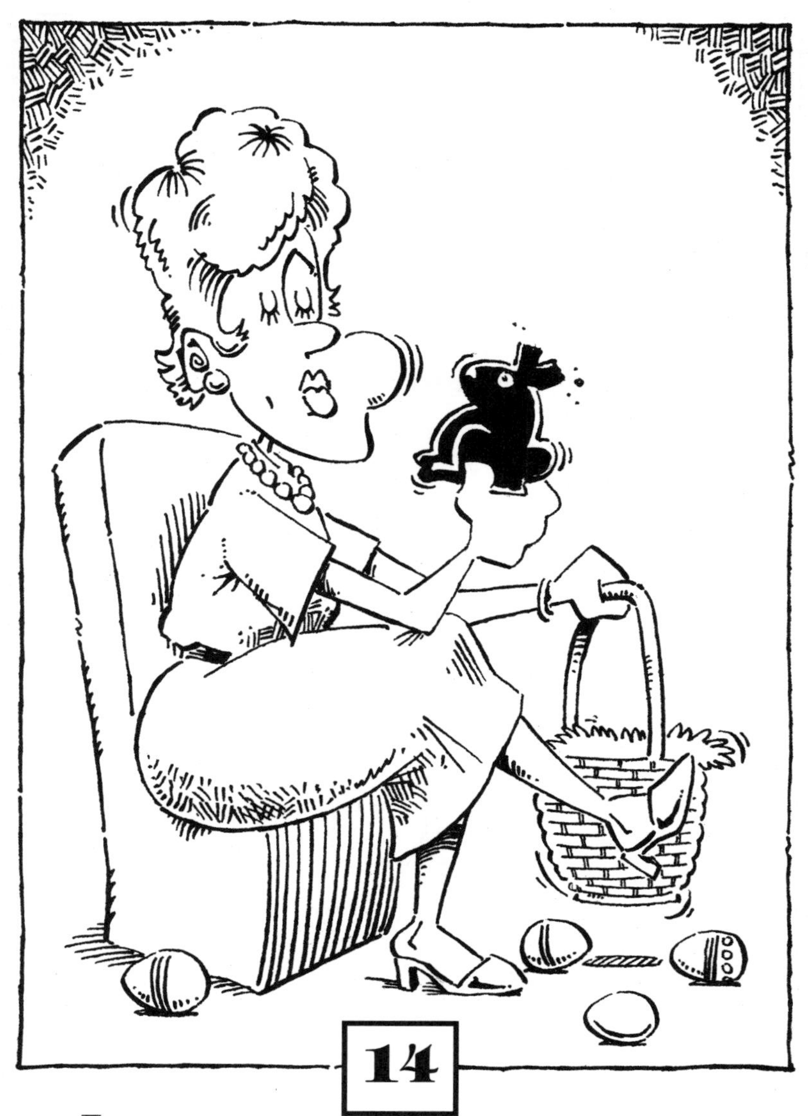

14

I still haven't finished the big chocolate bunny in my Easter basket.

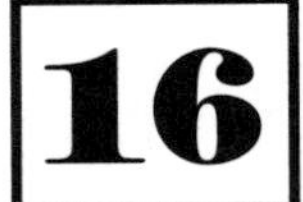

I'm having a mole removed.

I've finally gotten my couch
broken in just right.

17

The gym is too far away.

I have heartburn.

18

The whirlpool in the gym isn't working.

I've already lost an hour to
Daylight Savings.

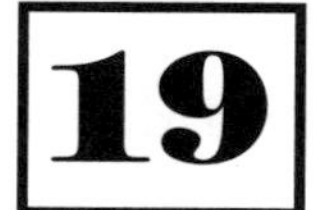

I think I'm anemic.

I might lose control of the remote.

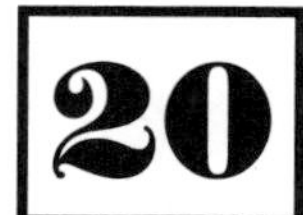

I'm preoccupied.

It's almost summer.

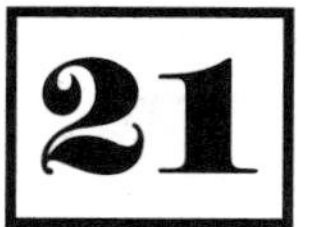

I broke a lace in my gym clothes.

The gym's out of my favorite sports drink.

My glasses slide off my nose when I sweat.

I tried working out before,
but I didn't like it.

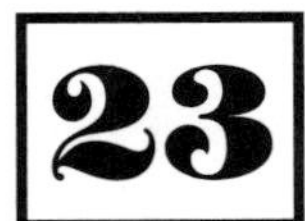

My gym clothes are all in the wash.

I've been thinking about it.

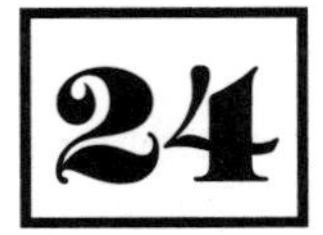

ARBOR DAY

After I get through planting this sapling,
I won't have the strength to
make it to the gym.

I try not to make any sudden
changes in my lifestyle.

The baby has colic.

I can handle my weight.

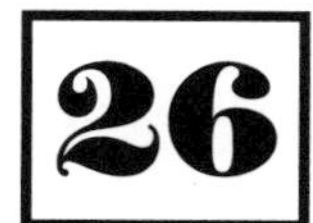

My hair is a mess.

My trainer and I don't get along.

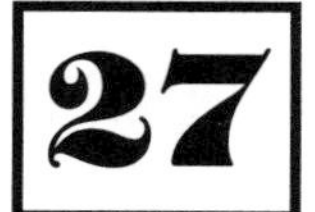

I would if I could, but I can't.

I don't feel like getting ready.

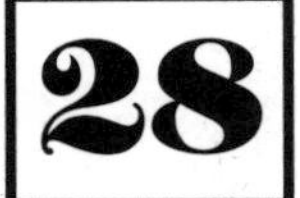

It makes me tired.

I ran out of gas.

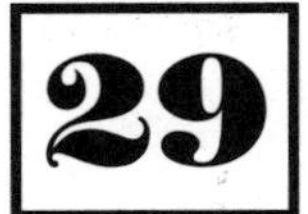

I might get a cramp.

I think I ate some bad fish.

It's too entirely too early for exercise.

I left my gym bag in the other car.

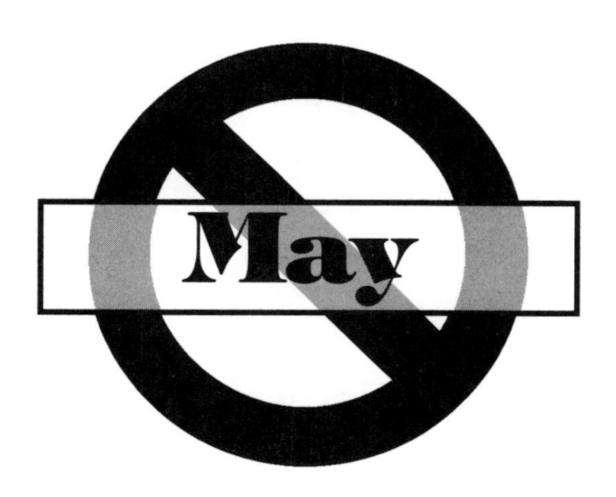

Point

"You still have time to work off those last few pounds and fit back into last year's swimsuit."

—Dana

Counterpoint

"The new suit you bought in April won't fit just right if you lose any weight now."

—Stacey

MAY DAY

I'll get my exercise dancing around the Maypole.

I just don't feel like it right now.

Tomorrow's a big day. I need my rest.

There was a power outage in the gym.

I do plenty of twelve-ounce curls.

My cat has a hair ball.

My two-week free trial membership is over.

I have belly button lint.

I walked enough at the mall.

They won't let me mount my portable fan on the exercise bikes.

I'm on the shake-a-day diet.

My seatbelt is broken, so I can't drive anywhere.

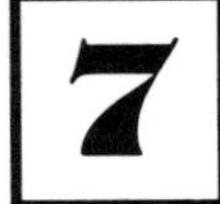

I have to plant my flowers.

I'd rather do cheese curls than weight curls.

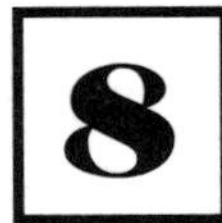

My chiropractor hasn't given me the green light.

I will when the gym turns co-ed.

I have to buy flowers for my Mom.

I have to take the kids to get flowers for my wife.

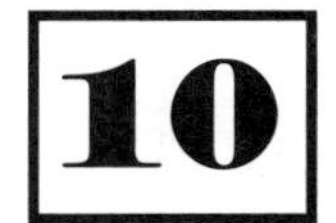

MOTHER'S DAY*

I cook, I clean, I slave. That's all the exercise I need.

I'm the Mom. You go work out for me.

My church is having a social.

I have shin splints.

I broke my glasses.

I'm going through a nasty divorce.

*Date changes yearly

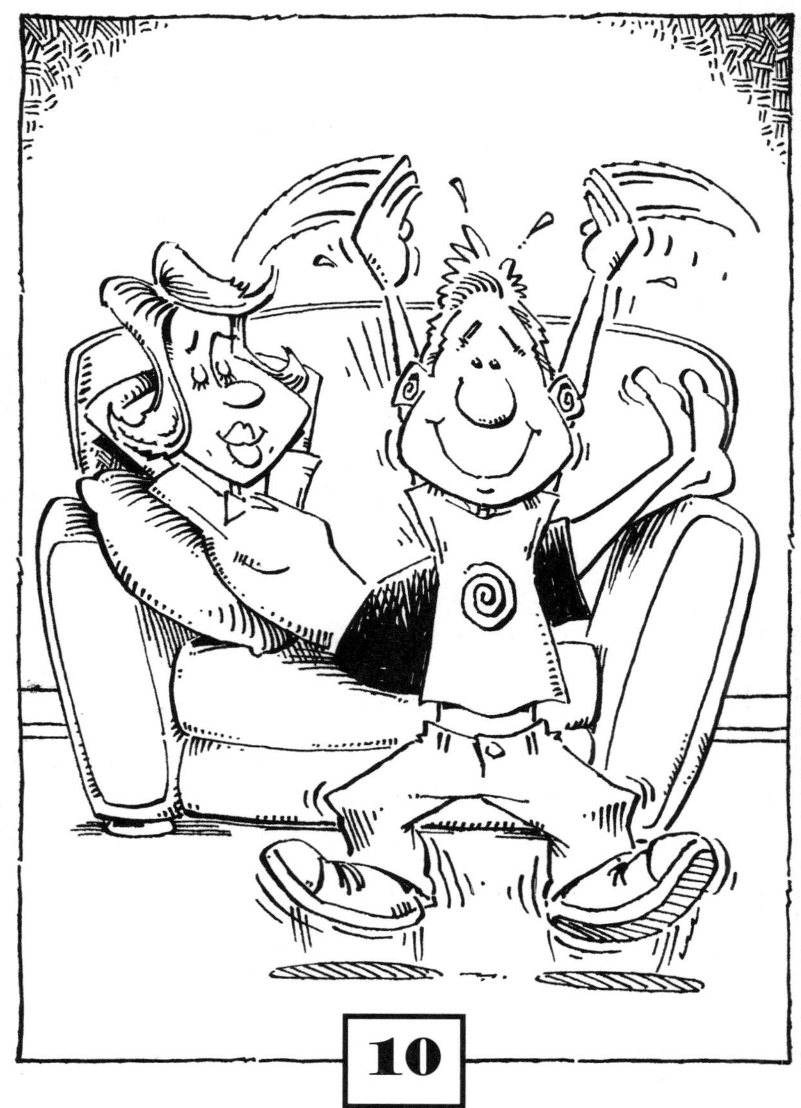

I'm the Mom. You go work out for me.

My gym just got hit by a tornado.

I just had surgery on my foot.

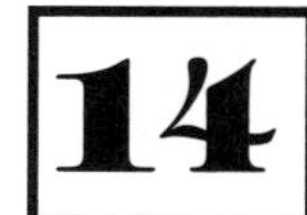

I will just before swimsuit season.

I have an itchy rash.

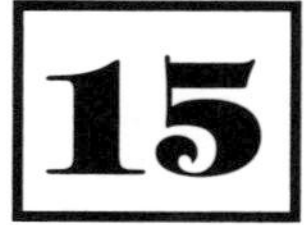

I lost a contact.

I can't keep up with the music in the aerobics class.

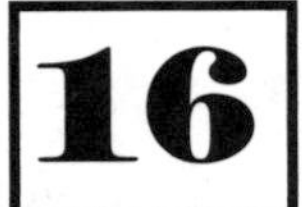

It's too nice outside to go to the gym.

I'm thinking of joining the Army.

ARMED FORCES DAY

I'm armed with a remote control.

If forced to make a decision, I'll choose walking at the mall.

I don't want my bust size to decrease.

I can't catch on to all those trick aerobic moves.

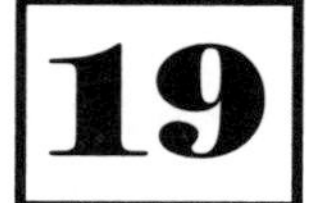

Gyms smell like sweat.

I have money. I don't need good looks.

I just had my navel pierced.

I'm taking the day off.

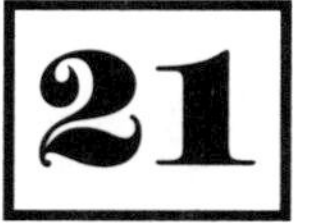

I might get a blister.

I'm having my wisdom teeth pulled.

I have to go to the bakery and pick up a cheesecake.

My dog's in heat.

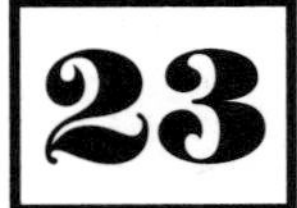

The second half of a made-for-TV movie is on tonight.

I have to download my computer.

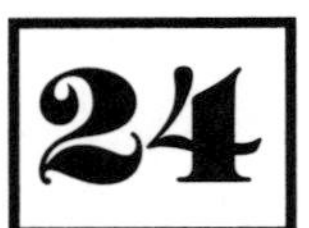

I have to renew my driver's license, and you know how long that can take.

I'm just getting over a cold.

MEMORIAL DAY*

I remember the last time I worked out.

Exercise is war. I'm a pacifist.

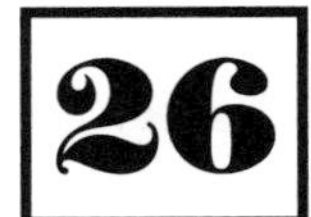

I would just die if someone I knew saw me there.

If I had more energy, I would.

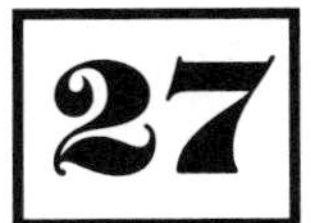

If I work out today, tomorrow I won't be able to move.

I'm listening to my new CDs.

*Officially observed

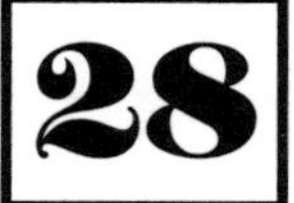

My knee hurts.

Gyms are too expensive.

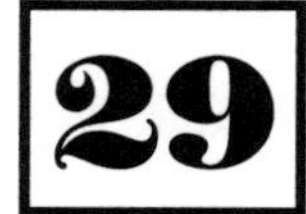

I have to study for finals.

I have a meeting with the boss.

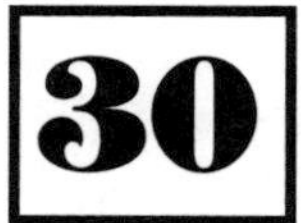

I think I'm getting emphysema.

It's too late.

31

I'm getting ready for a garage sale.

I'm too busy shopping for a wedding dress.

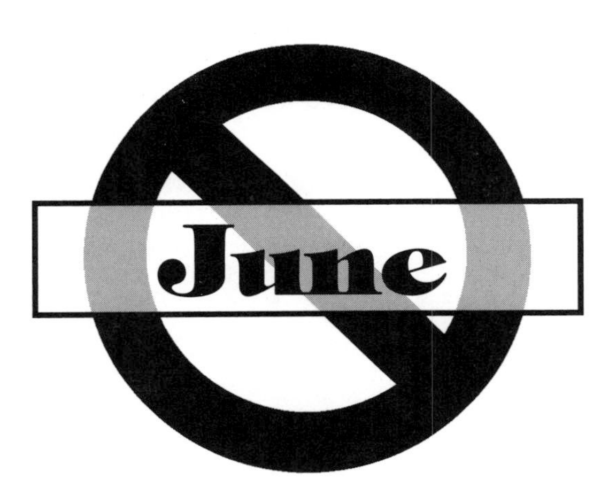

Point

"There are plenty of summer activities that include exercise. Playing Frisbee is a great way to burn some extra calories at a summer picnic."

—DANA

Counterpoint

"Laying out in the sun is a great way to break a sweat. And you don't have to lift a finger to do it! (Make sure you stretch out first.)"

—STACEY

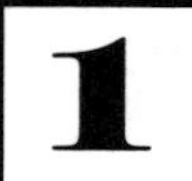

I forgot my shoes.

I've got to make a lot of calls today.

I have a doctor's appointment.

I have to give my dog a bath.

I'm working on my tan.

I don't have the energy.

I'm going sailing.

A week from Saturday I am going fishing.

I'm in a tennis tournament.

I'm too busy with golf.

My son has a little league game.

The club doesn't sell beer.

I promised the kids we'd go get ice cream.

I have to drive the golf cart for my boss.

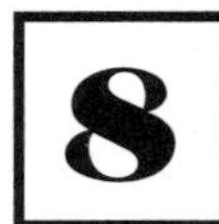

I have to pick out my Lotto numbers.

I'm stuck in Margaritaville.

I'm waiting for my Lotto numbers to be drawn.

I still haven't found the right gym.

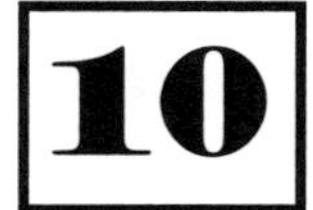

It's raining, and I don't have an umbrella.

I pulled a groin muscle playing catch with my son.

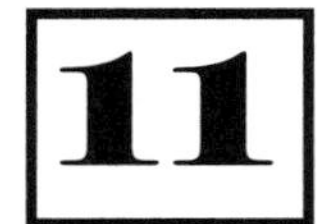

The water at the gym tastes funny.

It's my birthday.

I have tendonitis from using the mouse on my computer.

My membership expired.

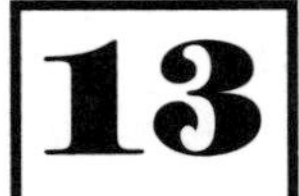

I need a bikini wax.

I have to wax my car.

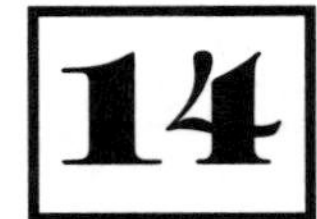

FLAG DAY

Horizontal stripes make me look heavier than I really am.

I broke a sweat just hanging my flag. I'm done for the day.

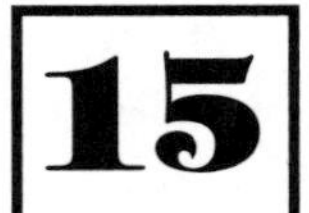

I have to clean up the house.

I have to wax my wife's car.

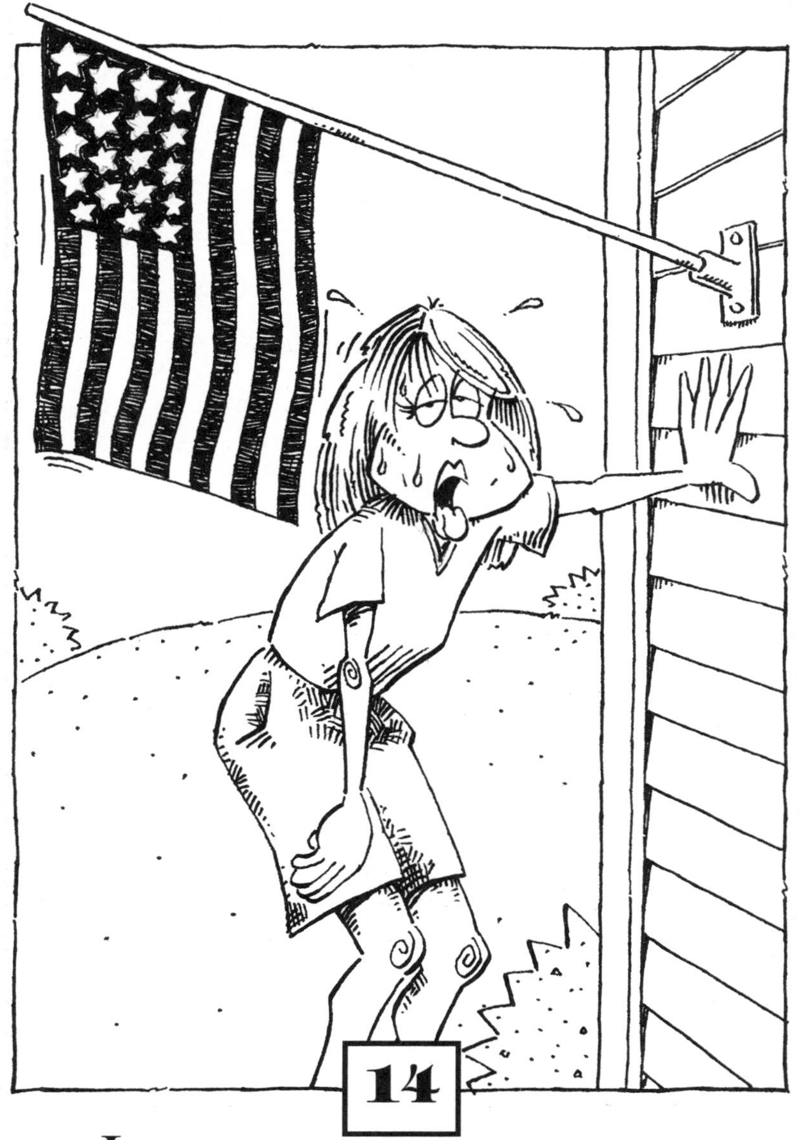

I broke a sweat today just hanging my flag. I'm done for the day.

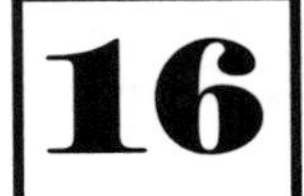

I'm getting ready for a beach party.

My hedges need pruning.

17

Spandex gives me a rash.

I lost something, and I have to find it.

18

It will mess up my hair.

I have to take the dog to the vet.

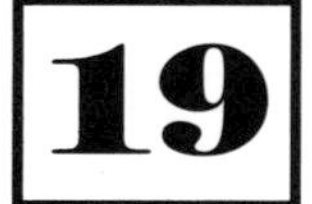

Sweat burns my eyes.

I get enough exercise at work.

I'm weeding the garden.

I stink when I sweat.

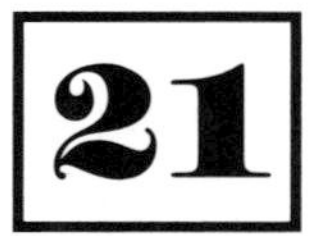

FATHER'S DAY*

Do you have any idea how long it takes me just to decide on a tie?

Shopping for power tools always wears me out.

*Date changes yearly

It's too hot in the gym.

I've been watching a lot of workout videos.

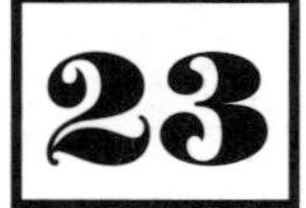

My legs will get too big.

I don't like it when my clothes stick to me.

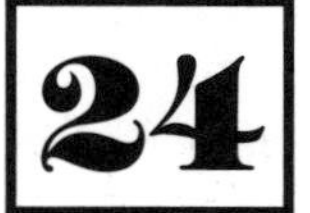

I have a splinter in my foot.

The check I used to pay for my membership bounced.

I need to dye my roots.

I think I look pretty darn good for my age.

I don't want my breasts to sag.

I don't want to miss the
hors d'oeuvres at happy hour.

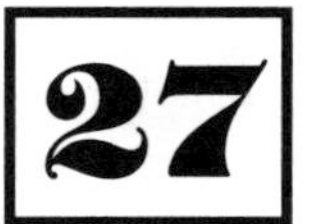

I have varicose veins.

I'm having a hemorrhoidal flare-up.

It's too sunny.

I have to floss my teeth.

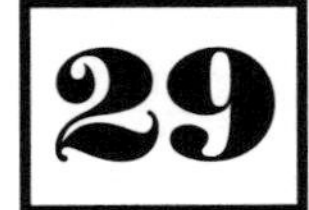

I might miss my favorite show.

I have to get to the bank before they close.

Macy's is having a one-day sale.

I'm having the septic tank flushed out.

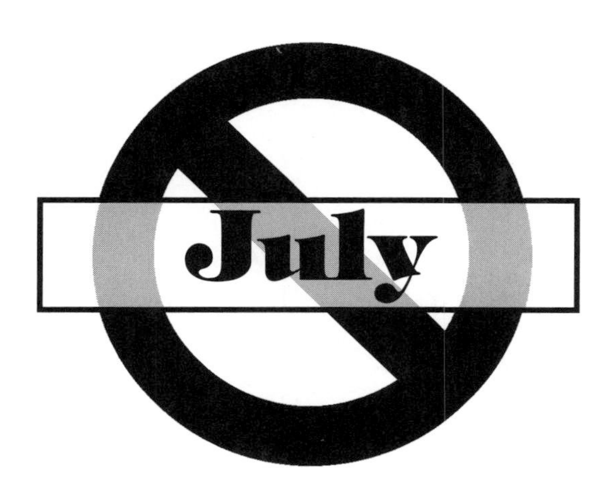

Point

"Take advantage of the beautiful weather to go on brisk walks in the evenings."

—Dana

Counterpoint

"Since your kids just left for summer camp, laze around in your quiet house and watch all the great reruns on TV."

—Stacey

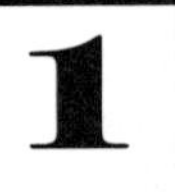

I have to work overtime.

I have no idea how to get started.

I have a party to go to.

I have to mow the lawn.

I'm getting ready for the 4th of July.

My beer will get warm.

INDEPENDENCE DAY

I'll sweat plenty standing by the barbecue grill.

I have the freedom to watch baseball games and soap operas.

I'm sore from swimming yesterday.

I'm worn out from celebrating America's birthday.

If I lose any weight now, all my stretch pants will look saggy.

I might run into my old girlfriend at the gym.

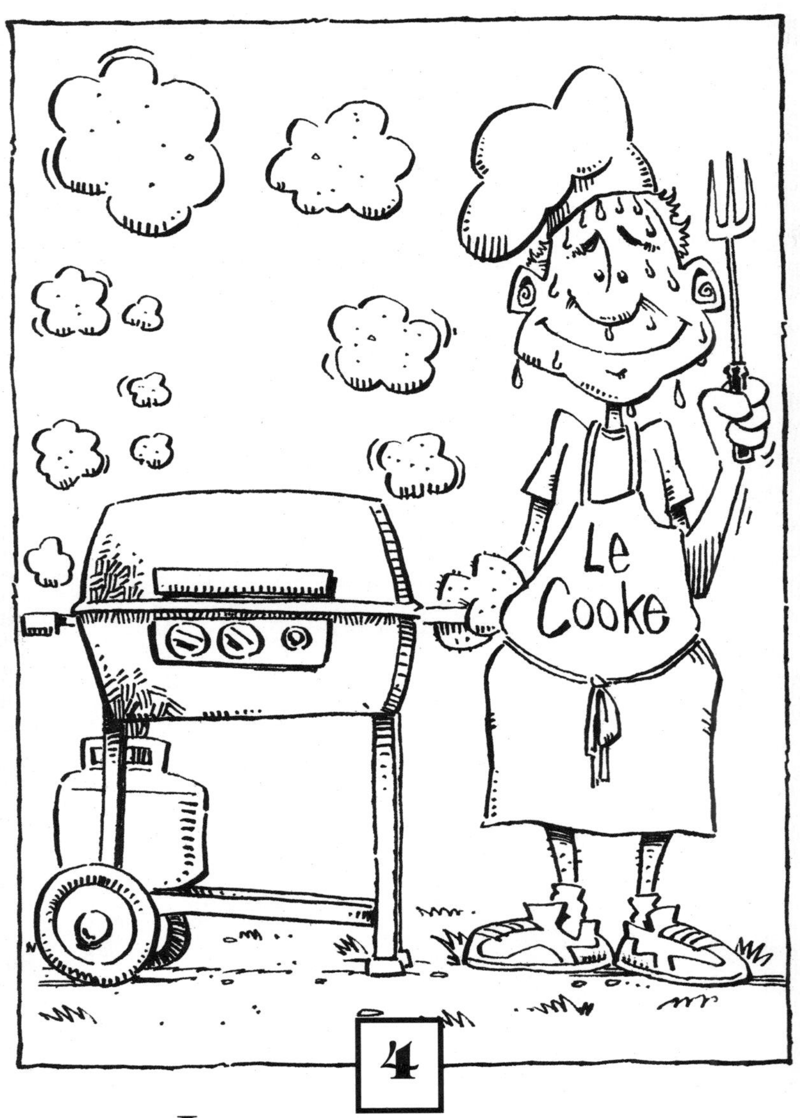

I'll sweat plenty standing by the barbecue grill.

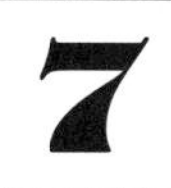

I'm moving.

I'm going to a barbecue.

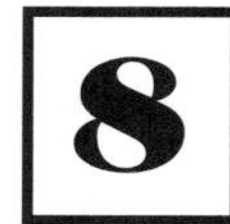

I'm going shopping with the girls.

I'm beyond help.

I'm planning my wedding.

I'm sunburned.

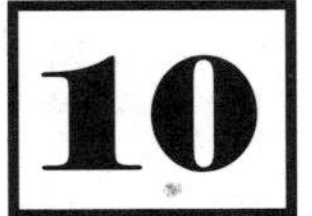

I'm allergic to Lycra.

My son has soccer playoffs.

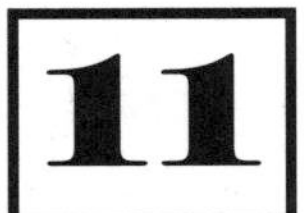

I could strain a tendon.

My kids are driving me batty.

I will when the kids leave for summer camp

It feels so good to just lie in the sun.

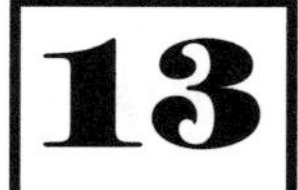

I break out when I sweat.

I'm suffering from heat exhaustion.

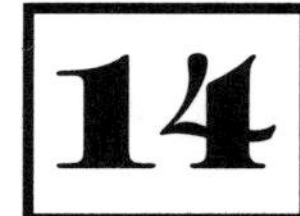

I have to weed the garden.

The trees need trimming.

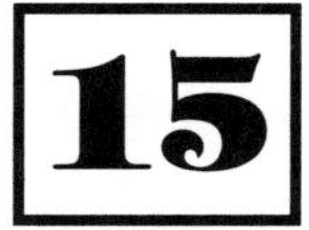

I just want to lay around and
relax this summer.

I'm repaving the driveway.

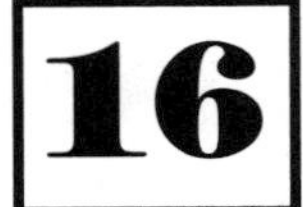

My vegetables are almost ripe.
I have a painful toenail fungus.

I'm not a morning person.
It's too hot.

I'm making strawberry preserves.
I'm going to the state fair.

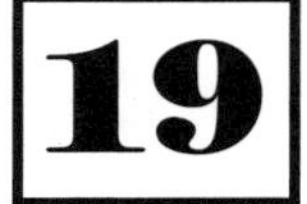

I might break a nail.

I have athlete's foot.

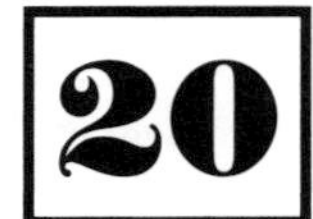

I have a major hangnail.

I just got drafted.

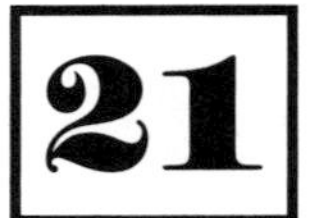

I'm taking a break from exercise.

I'm trying to clear up a bad case of acne.

My biorhythms are off.

The pool needs vacuuming.

My horoscope said to stay in.

I need to power-wash the siding.

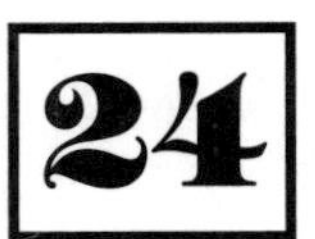

My mail was late.

They don't play country music at the gym.

I have a wart.

I worked out a month ago.

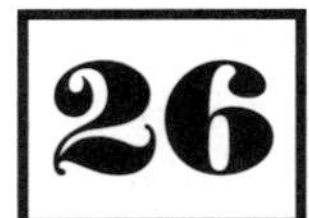

I have to take care of my sick grandmother.

I need a massage to loosen up first.

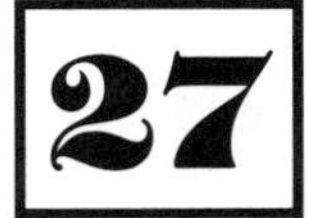

If I lose any weight, I'll have to buy a new fall wardrobe.

I have to make an important phone call.

I might get a blister.

I try to watch what I eat.

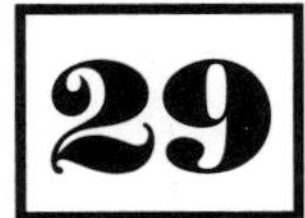

I just had my hair set.

I have to balance the checkbook.

I'm too old.

I'm totally depressed.

I'm too busy chasing the birds
out of my garden.

I hurt my back mowing the lawn.

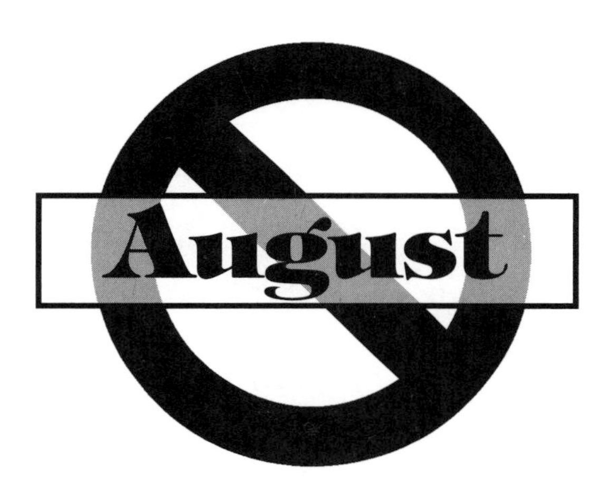

Point

"A lot of people make trips to the beach during this month. Sand-jogging is an excellent workout!"

—Dana

Counterpoint

"At the beach, having your kids bury you in the sand is an effective way to hide the weight you gained from too many hot dogs at summer picnics."

—Stacey

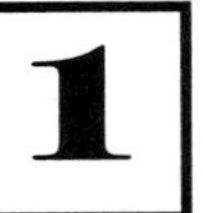

I'm planning my daughter's birthday party.

I ate garlic for lunch. I'd better not go out.

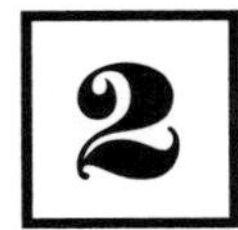

The trip to the wave pool wore me out.

If it's too hot, I'll just stay home
and eat fat-free ice cream.

I have to take the kids shopping
for school clothes.

Look, in this heat I'll get sunstroke
if I walk to the mailbox!

I'm dealing with a really bad case of poison ivy.

I can't reach the laces on my cross-trainers, and slip-ons aren't allowed.

My tomatoes are ripe, and it's time to can them.

I'll talk working out when I get paid big bucks to model sports clothes.

I have to pick up my voice mail messages.

I'm pooped from hanging up the hammock.

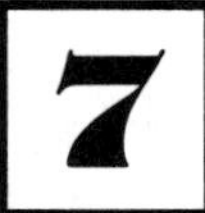

I have to respond to my voice mail messages.

I'm stuck in the hammock, and I can't get out.

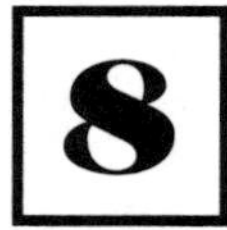

Lifting weights ruins my golf swing.

I've got to reprogram the channels on my VCR.

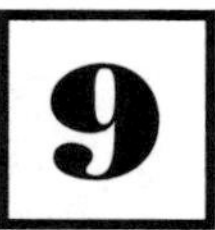

I have a million other things to do.

I can't find the lace to one of my tennis shoes.

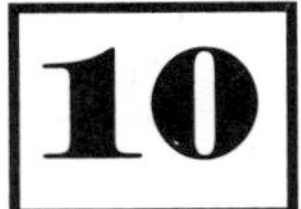

If I had more energy, I would.

Oh, like modeling agencies are going to flock to my door if I lose a few pounds.

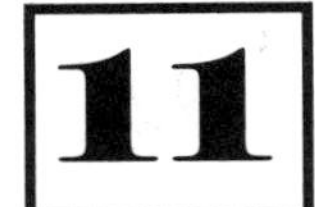

I'm trying to fix the lawn mower.

My pictures from vacation came back today.

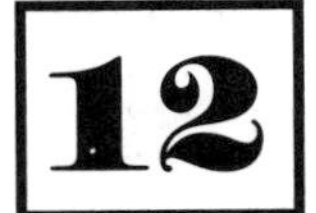

My computer has a virus.

I get hives when I'm around sweaty people.

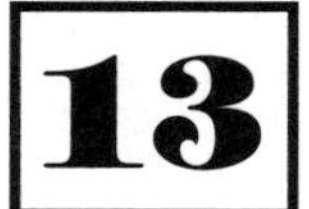

There is a really great end-of-summer sale at the mall.

People look at me funny at the gym.

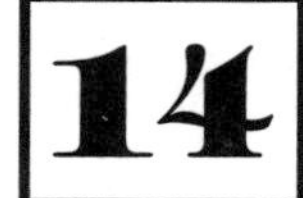

I'm watering the lawn.

Oh, no. Overdue library books.

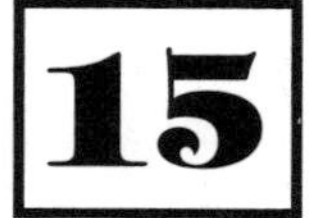

My sinuses are acting up.

My Jane Fonda tape is stuck in my VCR, and I need to take it to the shop.

My glasses fog up when I sweat.

I only work out on days when Dennis Rodman's hair is natural.

Today is my anniversary. I have to conserve my energy.

My gossip magazines are out on the newsstands today. Gotta go.

I switched to fat-free popcorn. Isn't that enough?

My wife gets jealous when I go to the gym.

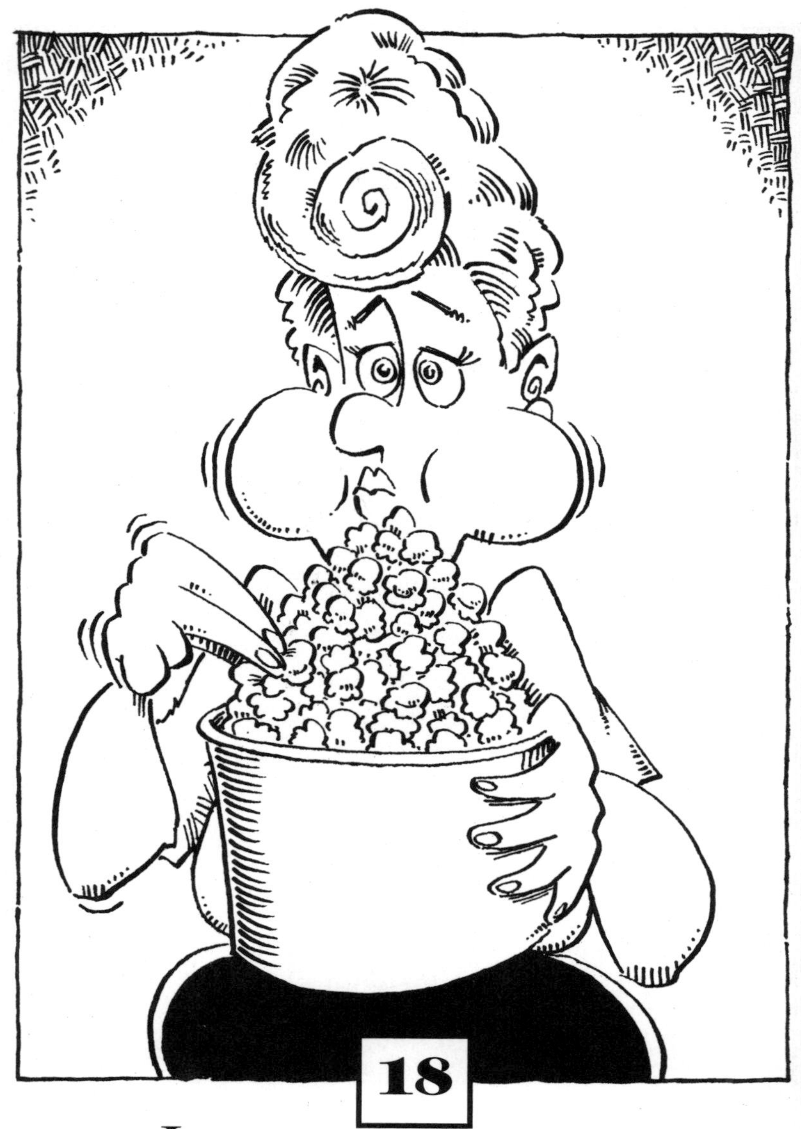

I switched to fat-free popcorn.
Isn't that enough?

Exercise makes my nose run.

I've started my own workout plan—
contract bridge.

I hurt my ankle trying to put the
cookie jar up out of my reach.

I just gave blood.

I get exercise. My convertible
has a manual top.

I have to pick up the kids from
summer camp.

My husband likes me the way I am.

We're going to a baseball game tonight.

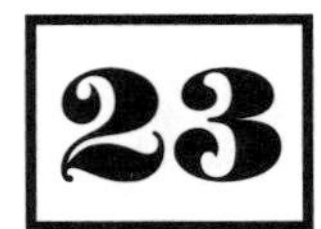

My boyfriend's sister's best friend's aunt died.

The time just slips away when I'm watching the weather channel.

My gym bag is being held for ransom.

I'm brewing beer.

I flunked gym in school, and I vowed never to put myself through that again.

I'm picking up my new car.

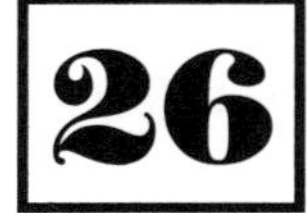

I'm in the middle of a good book.

I have an appointment with my stock broker.

I'm not the exercise type.

My cell phone doesn't work in the gym.

Join the health club? Hah! I'm joining the book club.

My psychic hot line has a special on this week.

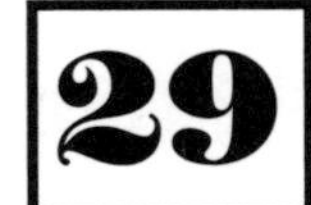

Those weights are too heavy.

I just don't lose much weight when I work out.

My children want me to spend more time with them.

I need to take out the garbage.

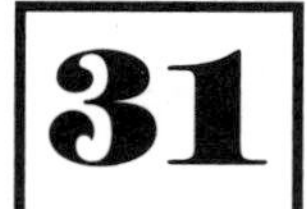

My daughter's hamster is on the loose.
My ulcer is acting up.

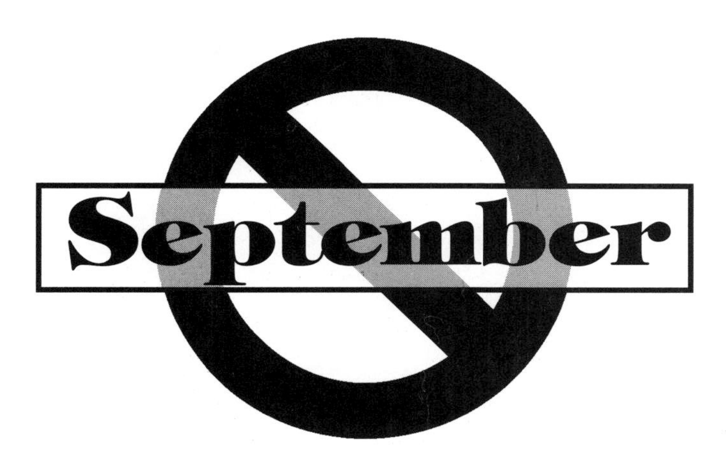

Point

"This month seems to be the 'Back-to-the-old-routine' month. Don't let exercise slip from your routine."

—DANA

Counterpoint

"Now that the kids are back in school, laze around your quiet house and catch up on all the soaps."

—STACEY

I have a naturally fast metabolism.

I'm going to replace the shingles on our roof today.

Doesn't work count as labor?

We're going to a church picnic.

It's my mother-in-law's birthday.

My therapist says that health clubs are bad for my psyche.

I've got to bathe the cat . . .
and the dog. Whatever.

We're having a family reunion. I'll get a workout just trying to remember everybody's name.

My porch swing is broken.

It's football season.

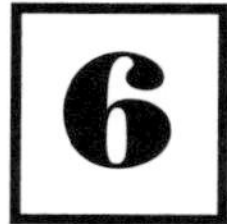

I'm still recovering from the birth of my two-year-old.

I'm waiting for the exterminator.

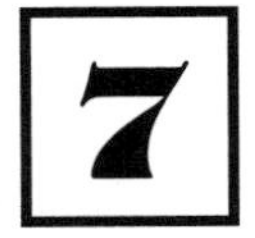

LABOR DAY*

Just thinking about exercising has worn me out.

When I'm not lying in the hammock, I'll be flipping the burgers. That's all the exercise I need.

My car has a flat tire, and I'm looking for a tow truck.

I have to coach my son's football team.

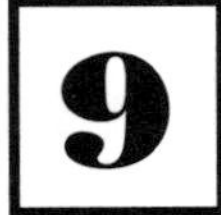

I'm exercising vicariously through Oprah.

It's time clean out the gutters.

*Date changes yearly

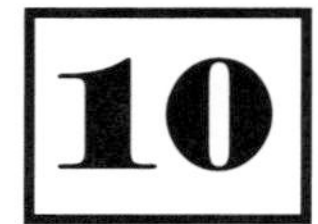

Look, I'm just plain antisocial.

I'm just not in the mood for that today.

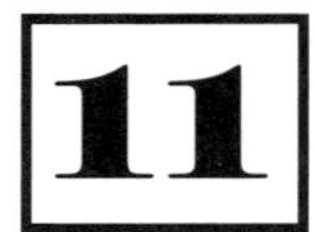

I have a bladder infection.

I need to spend more time with my wife and family.

The thought of fall and winter coming depresses me.

I have to help my son with his homework.

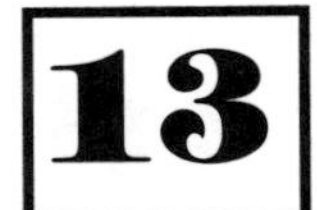

I've been taking the stairs instead of the elevator.

I'm bonding with my neighbor.

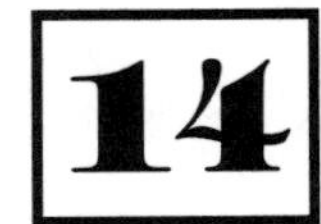

I get my exercise pushing the cart at the grocery story.

All my exercise socks are dirty.

I'm reading a book I couldn't get to this summer.

I have to hang out with Norm at the pub.

I locked my keys in the car.

I get bad acne when I sweat.

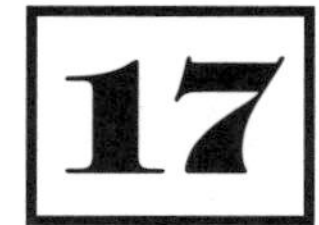

My daughter has a science project due tomorrow.

I don't like others who exercise. I'd feel like a hypocrite if I did.

I don't want to be vain.

The air conditioner broke in my car.

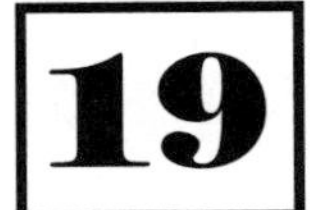

I'm really watching my diet.

I'm stretching my mind these days.

20

I have to go shopping for my winter workout clothes.

I'm really happy with the way I am.

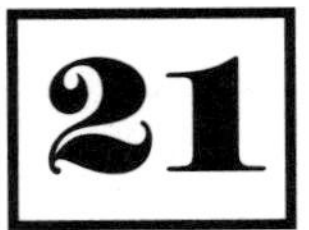

ROSH HASHANA*

I'm busy celebrating the Jewish New Year.

I'm studying for the bar exam.

*Date changes yearly

I have to take a shower.

I'm waiting for our new mattress and box spring to be delivered.

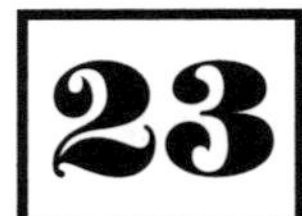

I don't want the new trainer guy to see me till I've lost some weight.

I've fallen, and I can't get up.

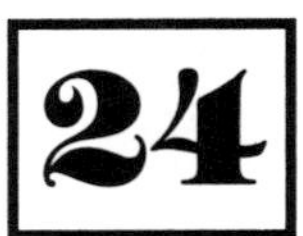

I'm healthy as a horse.

Where's the beef?

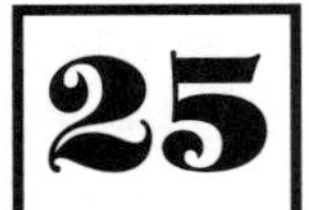

I've lost an earring . . . actually two.

I don't have the time.

I have to go to a wedding.

The doctor says I have to quit smoking first.

I lost my locker key.

I think my license expired.

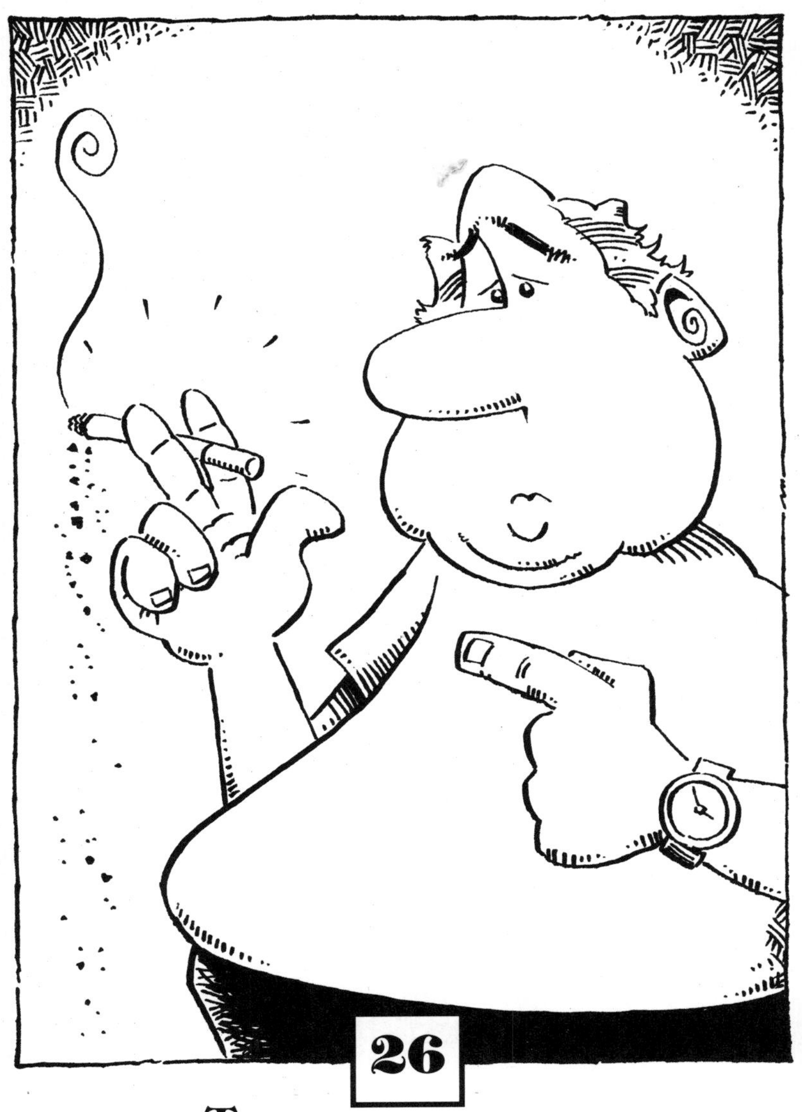

26

The doctor says I have to quit smoking first.

I have to help my daughter with her book report.

I'm working a second job to pay for the membership.

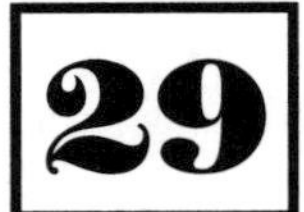

I'm way too tense to work out today.

I think there's a squirrel in our fireplace.

YOM KIPPUR*

I'm fasting today.

It's time to mulch the garden for next spring.

*Date changes yearly

We're thinking about remodeling our house.

My last workout took too long.

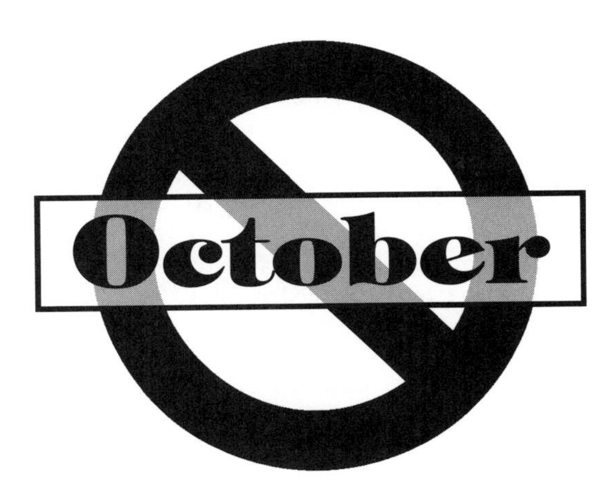

Point

"Since the weather is steadily turning colder, now's the time to bring your workout back to the gym."

—DANA

Counterpoint

"Colder weather means bulkier clothing!"

—STACEY

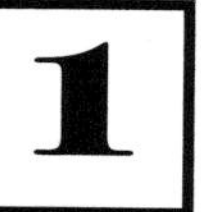

My neighbor is on vacation, and I have to get her mail.

I have to rake leaves.

I've got to clean out the refrigerator.

I want to watch football on television.

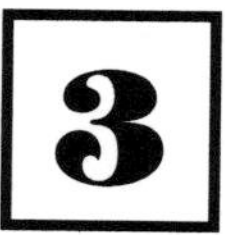

I'm trying to learn to speak Russian.

I get my workout jumping up and down watching football.

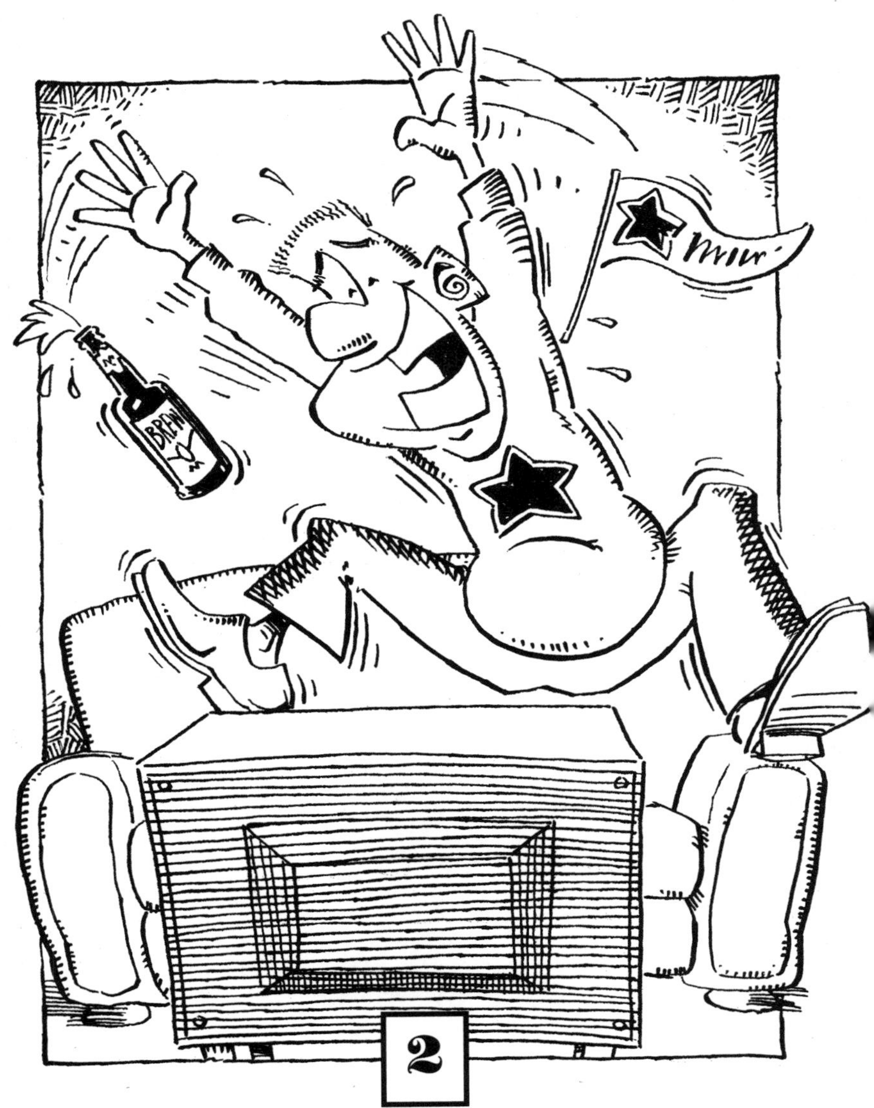

2

I want to watch football on television.

I'm having a yard sale.

We are going to the cider mill.

I go to another gym on Wednesdays.

I want to get an early start on making the kids Halloween costumes.

I'm afraid I'll become addicted to exercise and get too thin.

My mother-in-law is coming to town.

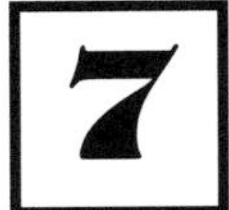

My doctor says I'm just fine.

I don't like it when my trainer tells me what to do.

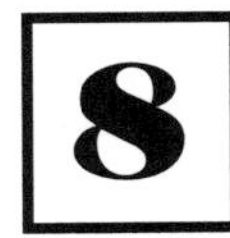

I don't want to miss the mailman.

I pulled a muscle raking leaves

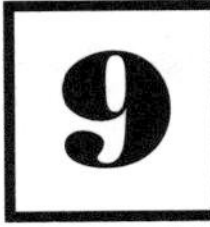

I'm potty training my two-year-old.

I have to bag the leaves.

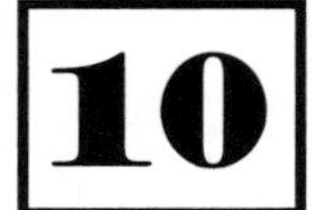

The club doesn't sell cider or donuts.

I've got an appointment with my accountant.

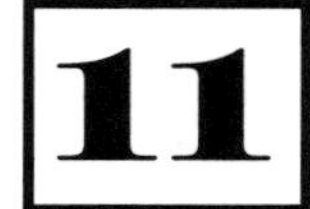

I'm not ready to commit to a workout schedule right now.

I'm having the TV repaired.

COLUMBUS DAY*

I plan to celebrate by taking a long soak in the tub, then beaching myself on the sofa.

I wish the world was flat; then there'd be no hills to climb.

*Date changes yearly

I get distracted by all the good-looking guys.

I get distracted by all the good-looking gals.

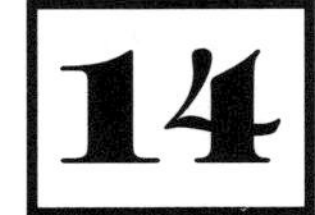

I'm going to the flea market today.

My job is very strenuous.

I'm picking the squash and pumpkins from the garden today.

Don't the stairs to the basement count as a Stair Master?

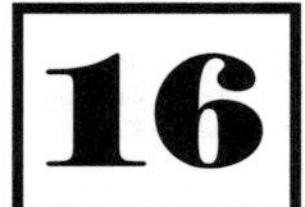

I just bought the thigh squeezer machine.

I'm under police surveillance.

17

Chewing gum has tightened the muscles in my neck.

I spent all my money on workout equipment.

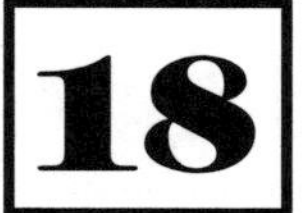

We have to pick out the Halloween pumpkin.

I can't find a sitter for the kids, or I would.

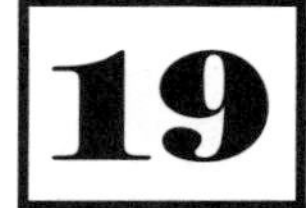

If I lose weight, I'll have to buy all new belts.

I just can't handle routine.

All the new fall clothes are out, so I have to go shopping.

The locker rooms are always a mess.

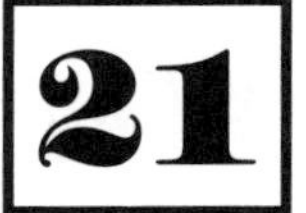

I'm having a tummy tuck.

I've moved, and I don't want to drive that far to the gym.

We have to carve the Halloween pumpkin.

Isn't today a holiday?

I'm learning needlepoint so I can make Christmas gifts this year.

I have to go to parent-teacher conferences.

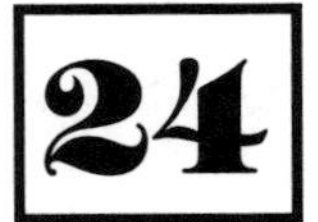

I'm planning my future.

I just got a new tattoo.

25

DAYLIGHT SAVING'S TIME ENDS*

Daylight savings time is over, and I want to sleep the extra hour.

I have to regrout the tile in the bathroom.

I get enough exercise just pushing my luck.

I get my exercise chasing my wife around the bedroom.

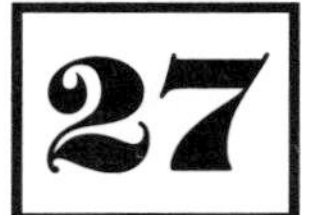

I need to get some more rest.

I have to get ready for a big meeting in the morning.

*Date changes yearly

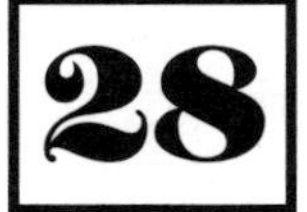

I'm allergic to my own sweat.

I just don't care about fitness.

I have to buy candy for the trick-or-treaters.

There's a storm warning.

A bunch of kids just egged my car.

I drank too much last night,
and I'm not feeling so good.

HALLOWEEN

I scare myself when I work out.

I'll just ride my broom around the block a few times to scare the trick-or-treaters.

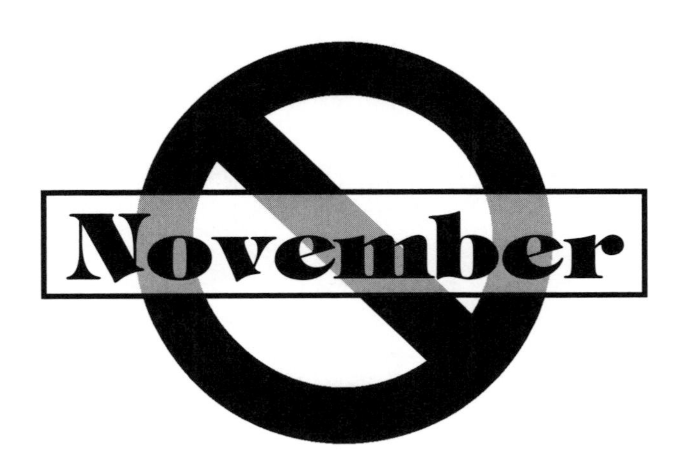

Point

Don't let the hustle and bustle of the holiday season get to you. Exercise helps to decrease stress."

—Dana

Counterpoint

"Shopping and baking will feel like a sufficient workout by the end of the day!"

—Stacey

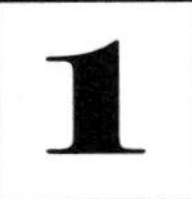

I'm still sorting through my kids' Halloween candy.

I'm going to get a flu shot.

I feel sick from eating too much candy.

My kids are sick from eating too much candy.

ELECTION DAY*

I'll get a workout standing in line to vote.

I vote for going out for pizza after I'm finished voting.

*Date changes yearly

If I switch from sugar to artificial sweetener, I can't help but lose weight.

My wife has a cold.

I sold my membership to the neighbors.

Deer season just opened, and I have to polish my shotgun.

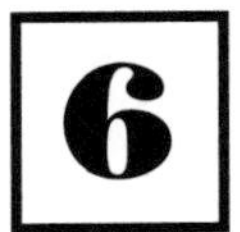

I'm having a hot flash.

My dog is having a c-section today.

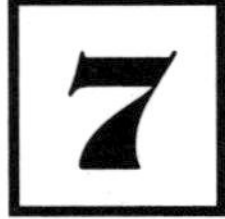

I have to get started on my Christmas shopping.

I'm going to a matinee movie today.

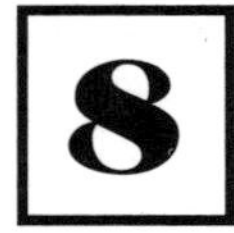

Don't I burn any calories watching those workout videos?

I hate all that counting.

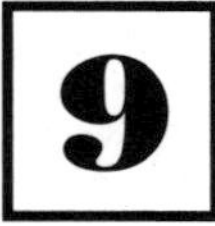

I am making holiday crafts.

Since I've gotten so heavy, exercise makes my side hurt.

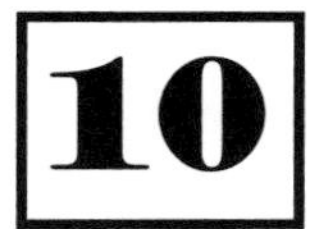

I have asthma.

It would be an insult to my wife's cooking if I lost any weight.

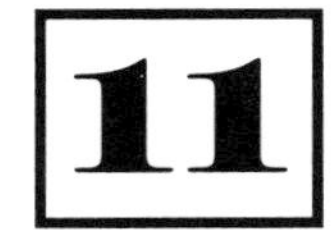

VETERANS DAY

I'll have to park three blocks from the parade route. That should equal seven hours on a treadmill.

I'll just walk down to the mailbox and put up a flag.

I need to spend the day making plans for Thanksgiving.

I've got to babysit for my sister.

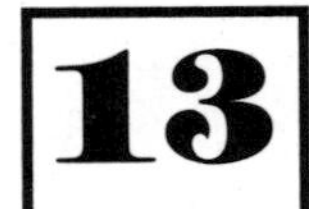

There's no place to clip my pager on my gym clothes.

The sauna at the gym is too hot.

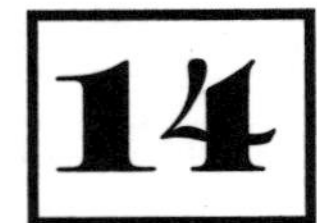

The sauna at the gym is too crowded.

My dog hates it when he sees me leaving for the gym.

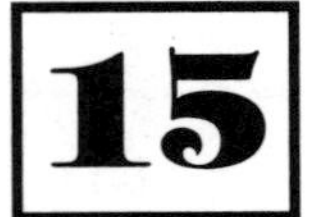

My head hurts.

I'd rather have a root canal.

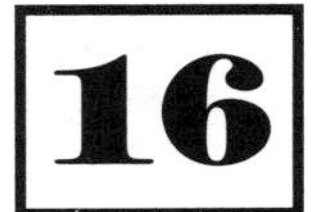

I don't like the music they play in the gym.

I'm programming the speed dial numbers on my new phone.

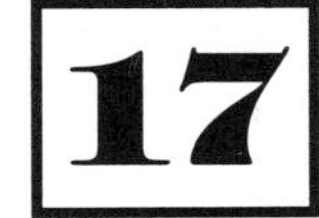

The trainers at the gym intimidate me.

My medication makes me dizzy.

I just got my nails done, and I can't take a chance on losing one.

I can't fit my lap-top on the treadmill.

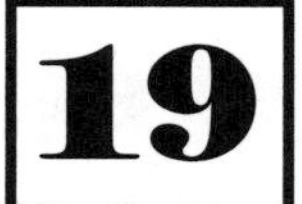

I'm getting plenty of exercise raking leaves.

It's time to put up the storm windows.

I was making pot roast, and
the oven exploded.

I won't have time to take a shower, and I
don't want to go outside in sweaty clothes.

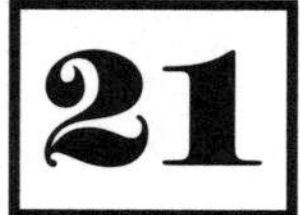

It gets dark too early this time of the year.

I'm too stressed out right now.

I have to make pies today.

My boss won't let me have a day off.

Thanksgiving is at my house this year.

I'm afraid I'll be the largest person at the gym.

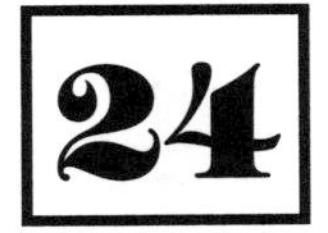

I pulled a muscle just bringing home the groceries.

I'm training my parrot to tell me I look like I've lost weight.

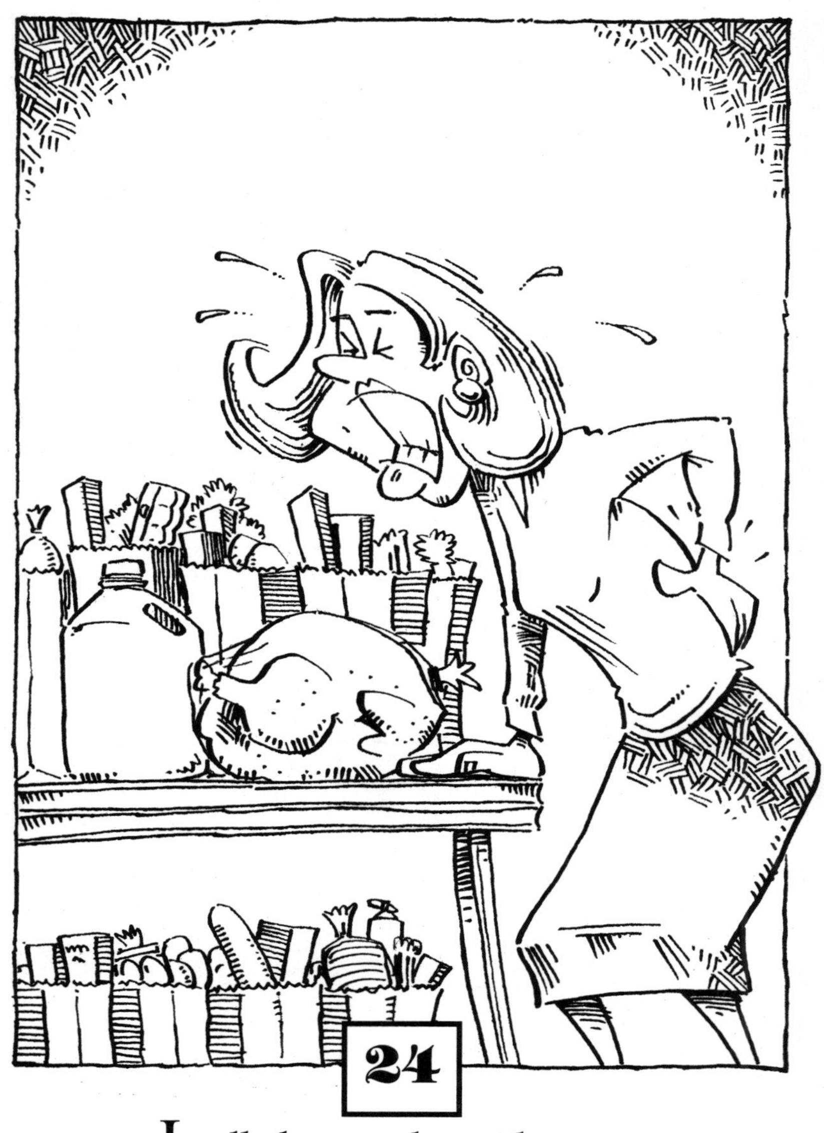

I pulled a muscle just bringing home the groceries.

I have to baste the turkey.

I lost a contact in the stuffing.

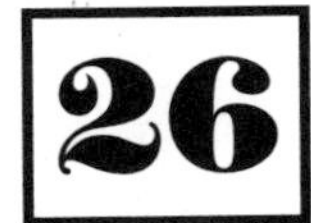

THANKSGIVING DAY*

I'm stuffing the turkey, then myself.

I'm giving thanks the gym is closed today!

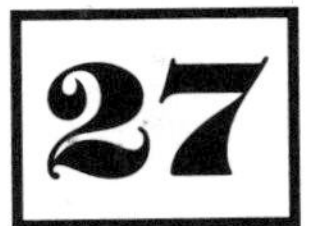

If I work out, I'll miss the best shopping day of the year.

I haven't recovered yet from Thanksgiving.

*Date changes yearly

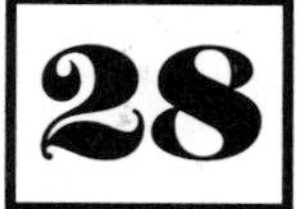

I need to rest from being jostled at the malls.

I can't do aerobics. I don't have any rhythm.

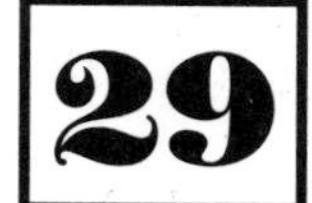

I'm afraid I'll see my ex and his new, young, blonde wife.

Both of my kids have basketball practice this afternoon.

I think we're going on vacation. This has been too much.

I have an artificial hip joint.

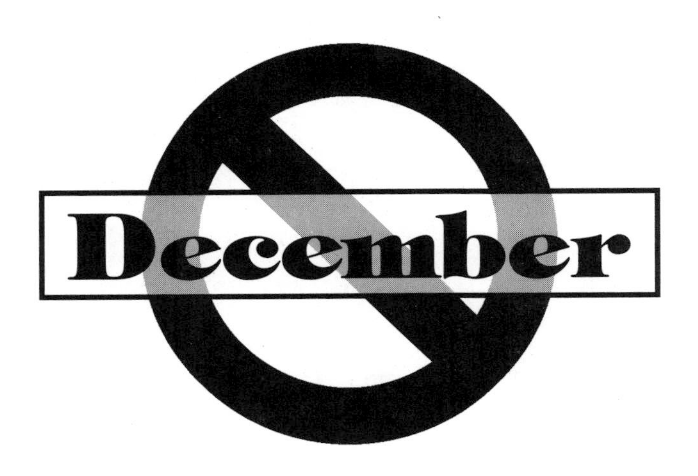

Point

"Compensate for holiday over-eating with frequent trips to the gym."

—DANA

Counterpoint

"Enjoy the holiday feasts, and put exercising on your list of New Year's resolutions—the ones you aren't planning on keeping anyway!"

—STACEY

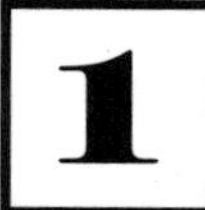

I still have lots more presents to buy.

I've got to return the movies I rented.

I'm making popcorn balls
and caramel apples.

I'm busy dreaming of a white Christmas.

I have to bake Christmas cookies.

I saw a picture of my trainer on the
bulletin board at the post office.

I ate too many cookies.

I slipped a disk hauling the tree into the house.

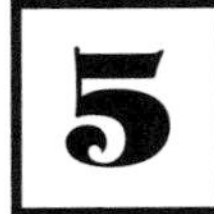

We're trimming the tree tonight.

I have to visit with the relatives.

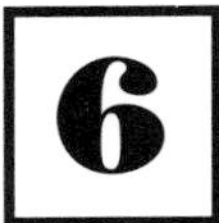

I don't want to miss the Christmas special on TV.

Everyone in my family is heavy.

I can't miss all the sales at the mall.

I went to the gym, but I couldn't get a parking spot close to the door.

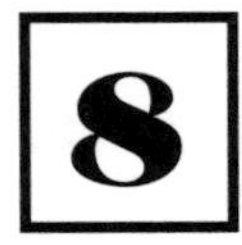

I'm still not done with the baking.

My bursitis is flaring up.

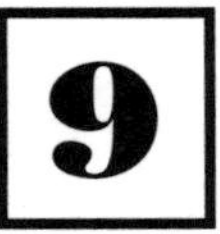

I've got PMS.

I'm going to start up again right after the holidays.

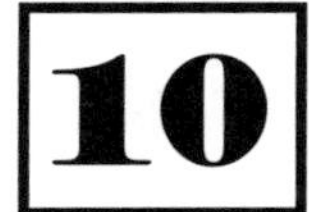

I've got to the grocery store before it snows.

I'm playing Santa at the mall.
I'm supposed to be fat.

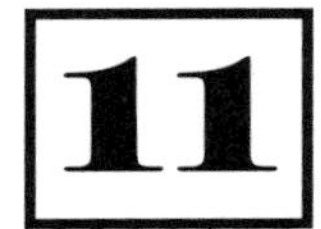

I have to buy a new dress for Christmas.

I'm afraid I'll see someone I know.

The gym is not on the bus route.

New Year is just around the corner.

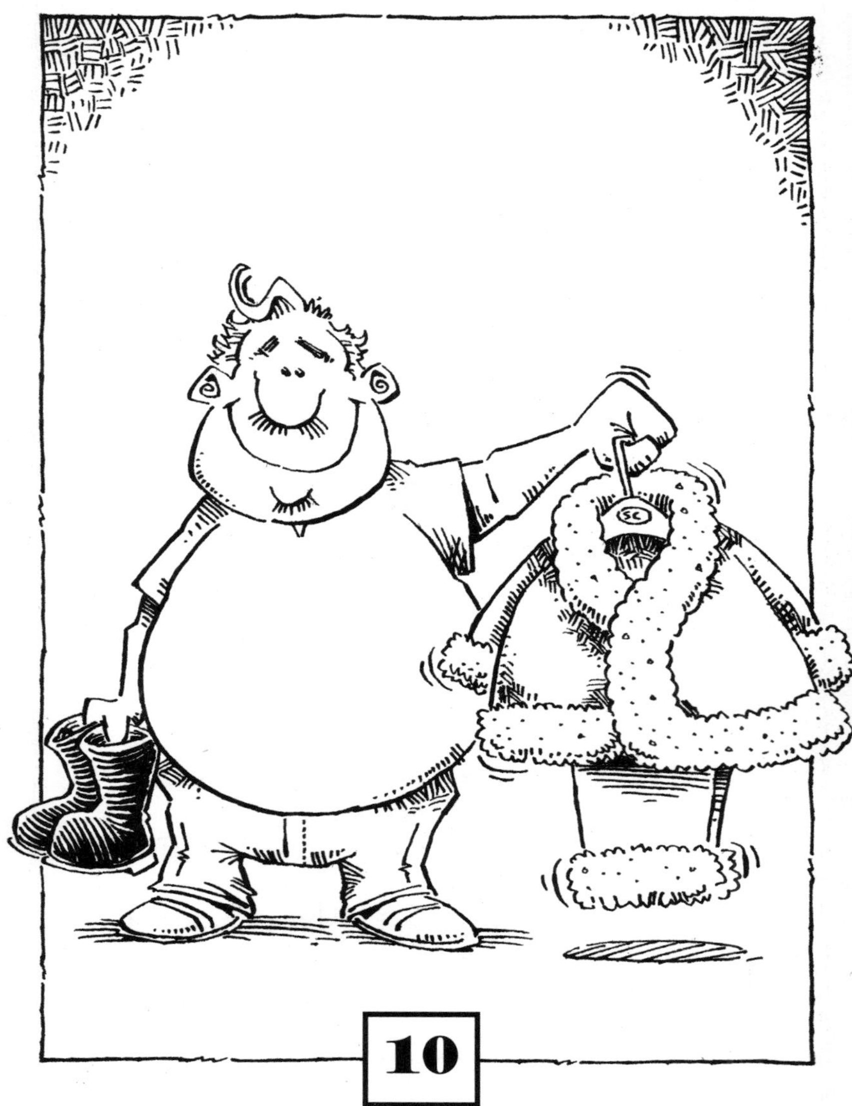

I'm playing Santa at the mall
I'm supposed to be fat.

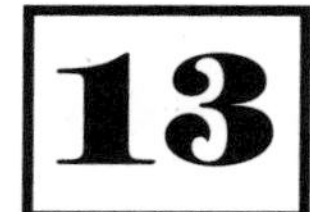

I'm still trying to untangle all the Christmas lights.

I have jury duty.

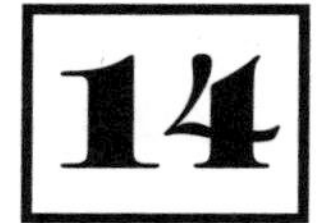

HANUKKAH*

I have to polish the menorah.

My office party is tonight.

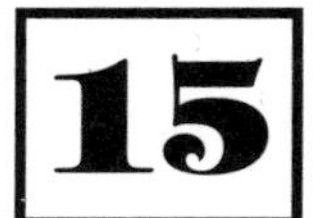

I have a pile of presents to wrap.

Exercise gives me a really bad headache.

*Date changes yearly

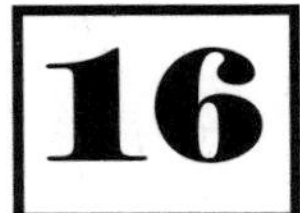

I've been invited to a wine and cheese party.

I slipped off the roof while hanging the lights.

I'm shaving my legs.

I asked Santa for a new body for Christmas.

I'm making the costumes for the Christmas pageant.

I'm cleaning my glue gun.

19

I'm going to say home and enjoy the Yuletide spirit.

I've got to take my Christmas dress to the cleaners.

20

All that sweating and showering makes my skin dry.

I'm tired from standing in line to see Santa.

21

There are too many mirrors in the aerobics room.

We are going caroling.

If I lose weight, I might look older.

I have an ingrown toenail.

I have to cure the ham.

I'm trying to select a long distance phone service.

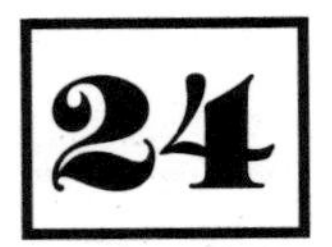

CHRISTMAS EVE

All that stretching to hang decorations has me whipped.

I've been wrapping gifts for hours. It's not all in the wrists, you know.

CHRISTMAS DAY

I'm spending quality time with the in-laws.

I burned more calories than usual walking back to the kitchen for seconds.

I'm exchanging Christmas gifts today.

I can't button my pants, let alone get off the couch.

I had a bad accident with crazy-glue.

I think I ate some bad food.

I started to go, but a black cat crossed my path and I came home.

The wallpaper in the bathroom is peeling.

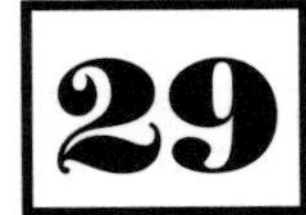

The new canary escaped from its cage.

I'm still trying to put together the Christmas toys.

I'm counting down till midnight.

It's one of my New Year's resolutions . . . I swear!

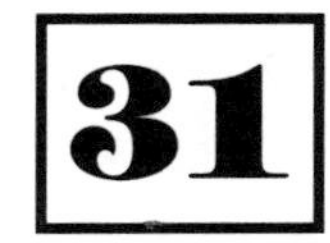

NEW YEAR'S EVE

I'll make a new year's resolution to work out at least twice next year.

I need to rest up for all the bowl games.

EXERCISE!

Twenty reasons to include regular physical activity in your lifestyle:

1. Strengthens the immune system.
2. Aids in reduction of pain associated with arthritis.
2. Alleviates depression.
4. Promotes weight loss.
5. Helps strengthen lower back muscles to prevent injury and pain.
6. Increases balance and agility.
7. Helps reduce blood pressure.
9. Helps maintain ideal body weight and composition.
10. Reduces the symptoms associated with extreme PMS.
11. Improves circulation to reduce blood pooling in the legs (i.e., varicose veins).
12. Helps boost metabolism.
13. Is an effective method for reducing stress.
14. Typically enables more restful sleep.
15. Increases flexibility.
16. Helps prevent many diseases.
17. Increases self-esteem.
18. Improves the quality of life.
19. Facilitates performing everyday tasks with less fatigue.
20. Lessens risk of premature death.

ANSWERS TO THE WORK-OUT APTITUDE TEST

5 points for every A answer
15 points for every B answer
25 points for every C answer

150-175 points
You are a fitness phobic!

Dana's Prescription: Start slowly, and don't be afraid. Make the right choice, and go to your nearest fitness facility to consult with a professional fitness trainer. (It is wise to check out their credentials first.)
Stacey's Prescription: Now you can't rush into these things. Give yourself some time to think it over and start slowly. (Suggestion: You may want to start with a few hundred massage sessions first.)

95-150 points
You're are doing the Fitness Hokey-Pokey! (You put the five pounds on. . . . You take the five pounds off. . . .)

Dana's Prescription: Don't be frustrated. I encourage you to continue to make healthy lifestyle choices. Be patient; it is a lifelong commitment.

Stacey's Prescription: Everything must be done in moderation, but don't forget to take time for the little things you enjoy . . . like, say, cheesecake.

35-95 points

You are truly a fitness enthusiast!

Dana Prescription: Keep up the good work! I encourage you to stay motivated, exercising regularly in moderation. Variety is the key. (P.S. Invite your friends and family to exercise with you, and have fun!)

Stacey's Prescription: My only suggestion for you is to memorize this book, carry it with you at all times, and start using the excuses whenever possible. There may be hope for you yet!